The Mythical Bill

sightline books

The Iowa Series in Literary Nonfiction

Patricia Hampl & Carl H. Klaus, series editors

Jody McAuliffe

The Mythical Bill

A Neurological Memoir

University of Iowa Press Iowa City

University of Iowa Press, Iowa City 52242

www.uiowapress.org
Printed in the United States of America
Text design by Richard Hendel

The University of Iowa Press is a member of Green Press Initiative and is committed to preserving natural resources.

Printed on acid-free paper

ISBN-13: 978-1-60938-154-7
ISBN-10: 1-60938-154-8
LCCN: 2012945878

FOR MY BROTHER, JACK,

AND MY DAUGHTER, MAEVE

One need not be a Chamber—to be Haunted—
One need not be a House—
The Brain has Corridors—surpassing
Material Place—

C. 1863, EMILY DICKINSON

I value my family more than my own life.

WILLIAM J. "BILL" MCAULIFFE

Contents

ETYMOLOGY: Torticollis, from the Latin *tortus*, past participle of *torquere*, to twist, twisted + *collum*, the neck: a condition of persistent involuntary contraction of the neck muscles, causing the head to be twisted to an abnormal position

Chronology

NOVEMBER 14, 1920: William (Bill) Joseph McAuliffe—Mc + Olaf, post-Viking invasion of Ireland, with red hair—is born, the third of four children of John H. McAuliffe and Margaret Cronin.

1926: William (Bill) Joseph McAuliffe, my father, undergoes a tonsillectomy at the age of six.

1942: My father enters the navy.

1944: My father develops spasmodic torticollis.

NOVEMBER 24, 1954: I am born.

NOVEMBER 25, 1954: One day after I am born, Harold C. Voris, Doctor of the Year in 1967 at Mercy Hospital and Medical Center in Chicago, performs radical surgery on my father for spasmodic torticollis.

NOVEMBER 27, 1954: Three days after I am born, my father threatens to kill himself and is committed to the psychiatric ward, 51B, at the Hines Veterans Administration Hospital, to which he is removed from Mercy.

DECEMBER 31, 1954: Bill is released from Hines VA Hospital.

1965: Bill begins to go demented—so-called "mental torticollis" commences slowly and inexorably.

JUNE 16, 1975: Bill is committed to Hines VA Hospital, Ward 51B.

AUGUST, 1975: William Joseph McAuliffe dies at Hines VA Hospital. Exact time and day of death unknown.

MAY 6, 1979: Brien J. McAuliffe, oldest son of Bill, is killed in a motorcycle accident.

Prelude

Bozo's Circus

What day is today, I hear him ask, my father, who is called Bill: the dreaded question. I've just woken up. Last night I stayed up late watching *The Yearling* on my portable TV with the rabbit-ears antennae—the one my mother let me buy with the fifty dollars I made dancing in *Sleeping Beauty* with the Leningrad Kirov Ballet. It sits on my desk so I can watch it from my bed. White gloves keep me from biting my nails to a pulp before I finally surrender, peel them off, and tear nails and flesh till I draw blood. That Jody boy in the movie loses his pet deer, Flag, but my beagle Star sleeps curled around my big feet on my parents' old double bed with the caning on the corners chewed out. My cousin Mary-Jo and I like to jump on it till the box spring crashes and my mother comes in screaming at us and pulls my hair. Late last night in the screen's flickering glow, I thought I saw Mr. McD, with his poodle Jo-Jo in tow, peering in my window trying to look at me—my room is just off the front porch—but I can't be certain. My dog will protect me.

What day is today? It's a simple question, simple enough to answer once, but not simple to have to answer a hundred times in the same day. Maybe if I answer it right away, the word Saturday will be the be-all and the end-all right here, right now. I mumble to him, Saturday, thinking if I don't make a big deal out of the question this will all go away, and then I head for the bathroom before he can ask me again. I'm afraid to look at his face to see if his eyes look strange the way they get when he's what we like to call "confused," without knowing the word used to mean "covered in shame." He works all week, then on the weekends he sometimes falls apart. He's not confused every

Saturday, but, lately, he's confused on more Saturdays than not. Usually, by Sunday he's not confused anymore; he returns to himself.

Do you want to have a cup of coffee with me, he says somewhat mechanically through the bathroom door. I detect a hint of desperation in his demeanor when I come out, even though the question seems normal enough. Maybe he's still okay. Sure, I say, even though fifteen is too young to be drinking coffee. It's something we can do together. I pour us each a cup and sit at the kitchen table, but I notice his place is empty. He's not sitting down; instead he's shifting his weight from one foot to the other in front of me.

Your mother's not here, he says. I don't know where she is.

I can tell he's afraid even if he can't articulate the fear.

I don't know how I got in this get-up, he says, tugging at his maroon velour zip jacket.

Why don't you drink your coffee, I say.

Okay, then, Jody, he says, all right then . . .

Now I know he's on the downward spiral. I get some Frosted Flakes and milk and try to eat. Everything tastes like paper and I start wondering where my mother is because I can't deal with him alone when he's like this. I'd like to get out of here, escape like she did, before it happens, but I don't know where to go. He disappears into the living room and I hear the TV playing low. I bolt the rest of the cardboard cereal and head back to my room to get dressed and hide out.

I hear him outside my door tapping. Jo, Jo—all I'm asking for is a little reassurance. Just a little reassurance. I open the door and he's holding the dreaded TV guide. Oh, well then, Jody . . . Come and see. We head down the hall for the living room, me following him. He shows me the TV guide and points at the TV. It's not the same, he says.

What's not the same?

What the TV guide says and what's on the TV.

I don't know, I say, and he looks at me as if the house is being lifted up by a tornado and spun around. I take the TV guide and look at it. I can see that the listing and what's on are indeed not the same. *Bozo's Circus* with Ringmaster Ned is not supposed to be on channel nine, but it is: the Prohut family of tumblers today. The father calls out for a round-off flip-flop and the littlest girl cries, I'll try, Daddy, and she does it.

They're not the same, I say. I point at the current listing and at the TV, confirming the channel. I sit on the sofa and he tries to sit down in his armchair, but he can't do it. He can't sit still even for a moment. Obsessing over the guide, he stands in front of the TV, looking back and forth between the TV, the guide, his watch, and me. He comes over to me and asks me again why they're not the same. I don't know, I say, starting to get short with him. When the TV guide and what's on TV don't match, he can't prove what day it is. I tell him it's Saturday; why doesn't he just believe me? Why does he keep asking me the same thing over and over? I'll try, Daddy, I hear one of the tumblers cry.

I have to do my homework, I say, as I brush past him heading for my room. My door doesn't lock, but he won't come in even though I can feel him hovering in the hallway. I just want him to go away or snap out of it and come back to himself. I hear him go into my brother's room. He tickles Jack's feet to wake him up. Thank God, I think, now I don't have to deal with him on my own. I hear him ask Jack the question, What day is today? I'm doing math homework and I don't understand how to do the problems. I'm getting really frustrated because I don't understand. First I start pulling my hair and then I start kicking the wall under my desk, but I keep trying to do the problems even though I don't understand them. The harder they are, the more I try to do them, the harder I kick the wall. After about an hour of this fun, fun, fun, I go to the kitchen and by now Dad is standing on the rug just outside the kitchen doorway. I'm experiencing difficulty in articulation, he says. How can somebody who's experiencing difficulty in articulation put together a sentence like that? That's why I half don't believe he can't control this breakdown. I'm having trouble swallowing, too, he says, but he keeps trying to do it—dry swallow—and struggles over and over till I yell at him to just stop doing it.

My brother is in the kitchen. He's three years younger than me. Dad tells both of us that all he wants is a little reassurance and asks us over and over what day it is. Sometimes we say it's Saturday calmly and sometimes we yell: IT'S SATURDAY! Either way it never gets through. I show him the TV guide and point at the TV, gesticulating wildly that there is a discrepancy between the two. I feel like a psycho salesman hawking television sets. There's a knock at the door. My brother and I panic. We don't want anybody to see our father like this. We have to get rid of whoever it is. Jack goes to the front door and I try to hustle my father into his room and out of sight. He resists with some force, though not yet all the strength he can muster. I have a few more hours before that starts. I push him back down the hallway and he starts moaning. All right then, Jody, okay then Jody, over and over. It's hard for me to keep him in his room because he's pulling on the door to open it and I'm pulling from my side to close it. Jack is at the front door with his friend Dave. The kids on the block want to play softball in the street out front and they want Jack to come out and play. Jack gets rid of him.

Jack's friend gone, I let my father out and he's more agitated than ever. I tell Jack to go ahead and join the game. There's no reason both of us should be stuck in here. He leaves and at long last my mother comes home from Great Lakes Naval Base where she's been shopping. My father is retired navy. She takes one look at my father and knows exactly where things stand. I leave him to her and go back to my room to study. I hear him ask her the same questions over and over and over. She yells at him and he moves down the hall to their room. I think maybe he'll go to sleep now. It's always better after he goes to sleep, even though (or because?) he can never remember what he said or did.

I put a record on my phonograph—*Rubber Soul* by the Beatles—snap on a pair of goggles, and sit under the sun lamp to try to burn off some of my zits. By the time I come out of my room, my eyes looking like sunny-side-up eggs floating in a sea of pink skin, Dad's in what we call his track suit—stripped down to his athletic tee and boxers and black socks. I don't know how he got in that get-up. Midafternoon and the boys are still out in the street playing ball. Dad's extremely agitated, looking like a rabid whirling dervish on the rug in front of the kitchen. He's beyond a place where any answers from me or my mother, in tones ranging from quiet to screaming, can reach him. She tries to move him from the rug and convince him to lie down. He wails in protest. I just want him to shut up, and all of a sudden he's on the phone dialing 911. He says he needs "outside help," whatever that is. My mother is trying to pry the phone out of his hands and hang it up before he gets the police over here. She roughs him up enough to make him drop the phone. I don't hold it against her. Then he starts crying and spinning in circles. He's on his way down now and he heads for the front door and out into the street in his underwear in front of my brother and his friends. He's running around in the street and the kids are all afraid of him but I can tell they think it's funny, too. My brother blanches. I don't know what to do, but I run after my father and try to pull him back into the house. I want to run away but there's nowhere to go.

My mother puts something on the table and we manage to force it down. I'm still hungry so I start eyeing my brother's plate. When he looks finished, I ask if I can take what's left. He nods and I eat that, too. It's Saturday night and I'm performing in *How to Succeed in Business without Really Trying* at the boys' high school. I'm playing Smitty and even though Miss Adrienne, the choreographer, told me not to sing Goddammit, voila in my song, *This Irresistible Paris Original*, I decide I'm going to do it anyway. Fuck her and the horse she rode in on. It's a Catholic school so she doesn't want me to sing Goddammit, but oh, dammit instead. There's a cast party afterward and I've secured a bottle of champagne ahead of time and planted it in the backyard for safekeeping. My friend, Marian, and I have been planning for weeks to get drunk at the party. It will be my first time. After the show, I spend the evening at this party in somebody's basement next to the dryer, leaning against a post, drinking the entire bottle by myself, getting dizzier and dizzier. At the end of the night, we get a ride home from two guys on the swim team a year ahead of me, one of whom will turn out to be my friend for life (the boy my father names the mythical Dan, because he never actually lays eyes on him), but I don't know that at the time. They drive us to my house and I have to stop the car several times on the way home to open the door in order to puke. On one of these numerous pukings, my wallet falls out of the car and into the gutter, along with all the money I've collected from schoolmates for tickets to see American Ballet Theater downtown. I don't notice a thing. They drop me off after midnight.

Did you lose something, my mother says, waking me up with a knowing smile. I decide to play it cool—I have no idea if I lost something because I can't remember much of what happened last night. She laughs as if it's all some kind of in-joke, a rite of passage, and tells me a lady from Oak Park called to say she found my wallet in a gutter in front of her house with 150 dollars in it. I must have a guardian angel. I believe in God even though I've stopped going to church, because I'm sick of those nuns telling me how bad we all are and giving us the silent treatment. My head is splitting and my mouth tastes of vomit.

I stumble out of bed and catch sight of my father lying on the bed in his room. He's neatly dressed and holding a rosary in his hands. I stick my head in the door and he looks at me with sad eyes, his real eyes. He says, I know something terrible went on yesterday, but I can't for the life of me remember what.

Are you okay, he says.

No, I say. I don't know. Yeah. I have a matinee today.

Knock 'em dead, he says.

I'll try, Daddy.

Part One

Diary of William J ["Bill"] McAuliffe [final entry]

Thursday December 19 [1974]

I just recently returned from my second stay at Passavant where I was taken + put in restraints because I put on such an exhibition that I went out of control + Joy had to take me to the hospital where for good or evil as far as I know I was running around outside in my pajamas + accosting various neighbors. I was in the lock ward there for some time having considerable difficulty swallowing + eating. This was gradually counteracted but not before a lot of anxiety + mental anguish. Even after being transferred to Ward 10 East I had an awful lot of terror + anguish. I've been even more terrified since I came home. Everybody insists that I must have something I enjoy doing as a sideline. I tried the clarinet but it's too difficult as I don't know all the sharps + flats + have forgotten some of the fingerings. I am trying to do some writing now in an attempt to reconcile some of these insuperable deluges of depression + despair that I'm feeling. As far as doing things that I like to do I'm writing now to overcome some of these feelings now that I'm home again. Honest to God though I don't know if I'll be able to hack it or not. God help me if I don't though, because this is the last chance. I always feel though that I'd feel better off dead. Well so much for now though.

WJMcAuliffe

The Great Escape

He called me Johannesburg, South Africa. They named me Johanna Dianne after my patron saint, St. John of the Cross, but only in order to call me Jody. Or, in his case, Johannesburg. Walking with him to church some Sunday when I am still pretty little, holding his hand, I take big steps to keep up with him, mainly looking down and assiduously—one of his key words—avoiding the cracks in the sidewalk. Step on a crack, break your mother's back. At that point I may have wanted to; she was my chief competition. Cut to Church of the Divine Infant in the western suburb of Chicago where I grew up, and we're sitting behind two kids younger than me, craning their necks around to stare at my father. I see them and so must my father but we say nothing. They will not turn away. I don't understand why they stare because I don't understand that there's anything wrong with my father. I don't feel ashamed. Erving Goffman, "a student of the problems of face-to-face interaction," would say that I was "a wise person." As the daughter of the torticollitic, I live inside his world, even now, long after he is gone.

In his *Manual of Diseases of the Nervous System*, W. R. Gowers applies the term torticollis to a condition in which contraction—persistent shortening or active spasm—of the muscles of the neck causes an unnatural position of the head. The condition, Gowers believes, is nervous in nature. There are those who see the metaphor quite clearly: the sufferer is turning away from something he does not want to see. The body betrays the feelings of the sufferer. The neck is in revolt, fear made visible.

My father had torticollis, even though he had surgery for torticollis on November 25, 1954, the day after I was born. His head and neck had come to an agreement without his knowledge. My current question of what exactly torticollis is turns out to be a good one because it is one of those questions that cannot be answered simply. I have a creeping consciousness of a certain symmetry, some as-yet-obscure relationship between his surgery of November 25, 1954, and my birth the day before.

He died thirty-four years ago. The date is in question. By the time the VA hospital decides to show his body to my mother, who is a registered nurse, she can see that he has already been dead for twenty-four hours. You're not supposed to die in the psychiatric ward. Your wife is not supposed to see your dead body twenty-four hours after the fact.

I am the same age as my father when he died. Why did he die?

Though I've never been in an actual war zone, my father certainly had. And though, or perhaps to some extent because, he never talked about it, the war colored my existence in ways that only now I'm beginning to understand. The truth is that I do not know what happened to my father—mentally, physically, or both. I do know that when I am ten years old, he sits me on his lap in his big red leather chair—the one with the telltale burn scars from when he fell asleep with a lit cig in his shaking hand—and he tells me that he is going to die in ten years. Why is he telling me this? And how does he know? Spasmodic torticollis is not a fatal disease. My younger brother Jack cites the cig burns in the chair as early evidence of cognitive decline.

I have to ask Jack, the only other survivor of my immediate family, what day my father died because I can't remember. My brother always seems to possess a precise grasp of the fine details concerning my father's life and death, whereas my narrative seems hopelessly quagmired in myth. Is the date of his death a memory that's been crowded out in order for me to remember something more important, and if this is true, what is it that's so important that I'm supposed to remember? I think I know my father died around the time of my mother's birthday—August 24—but I can't remember exactly. My younger brother suffered longest of the three of us children to witness/survive, in a manner of speaking, firsthand, the "bitter mercies" (quoting Bill) of Bill, who loves language, especially oxymorons. Actually, my father uses the phrase primarily concerning being left to my mother's "bitter mercies"—home alone with Joy, efficient employer of what he calls the kick-punch method—my mother, a.k.a. Big Nurse, so-named by my brothers and me after the merciless Nurse Ratched from *One Flew Over the Cuckoo's Nest.*

My mother, given name Mercedes, is convinced that if my father eats something he will not descend into one of his so-called-by-him "spells." She developed and perfected the kick-punch method to plant and keep him at the kitchen table where she could get some food in him. Though my father remained what he called "the titular head of the family," he was the first to admit, his eyes brimming with tears of laughter, that nevertheless, my mother was the one with the tits. Former lifeguard who hated swimming, great legs and built like a brick shithouse, she could keep him in his place, but only up to a point.

The question of who suffered/suffers the most—my father, my mother, me, or my two brothers—doesn't really matter in the end. Suffering is a quality, like mercy, that cannot be measured except, perhaps, in the degree of its bitterness.

November 19, 1972

Dear Jody,
I realize this is a little bit silly, writing you when you'll be home Wednesday, but I just wanted to add a few joyous moments to your otherwise cheerless existence.

Yesterday was a most peculiarly devastating day for me; started out with me playing the whirling dervish routine in the morning + ended with Joy throwing walnut shells at me in the late evening. Really a gung-ho day all around.

However, today I am fully recovered, I think. Brien came home yesterday for his birthday + is going back today. Well next Friday is your big day + I'll be home to help you celebrate in my most restrained manner.

Hope your play [Yeomen of the Guard] *went well this afternoon weekend. We'll probably be seeing you in it December 1st + 2nd, circumstances, of course, permitting.*

I love you, dolly, + hope to see you Friday.

Love,
Dad

The holy card for his wake says August 26, 1975, two days less than exactly thirty years before my mother dies on her eighty-fourth birthday, August 24, 2005. I remember precisely that he "expired"—the word my mother uses when she calls my older brother, Brien, and me at his house in Santa Cruz. Expire as in *exspirare*, *ex*, out + *spirare*, to breathe. In dying he could finally breathe—out. He would be pleased that I'm looking it up; that's what he says every time I ask him the meaning of a word—Look it up! This is why the dictionary is one of my favorite books—one of his many gifts to me, which include the mystery of his disease.

My mother had given me the impression that he had died of heart failure. I came up with the idea that his heart failed because the doctors overlooked the fact that he was dying of an underlying medical condition and placed him on the psychiatric ward. This particular narrative of his demise plays to my desire to believe that he had decided to die, because he had reached the end of the road with all tolerable options exhausted: a kind of justifiable, psychogenic suicide. In his desire to die, he stopped his heart. There is something powerful and ascetically romantic about this version of reality. Jack informs me that he essentially drowned—as did my mother essentially drown from idiopathic pulmonary fibrosis—from pneumonia in the psychiatric ward of a VA hospital, "crying" (my brother's word) that he wanted to be aspirated. He knows this because my father had been crying to him about it, before he was moved from the medical ward to the psych ward. The nurses were tired of his "spells" and tired of listening to him cry. They had lost the will to perform the task of aspiration, especially for some nutcase who belongs on the psych ward. As a result of this lapse in adequate care, and his having been in the wrong ward at the wrong time, he had inadvertently expired.

My heavily romanticized version of Bill's death scene has, until recently, exonerated me from imagining his actual death. In idle moments the images steal into my consciousness like a horror movie—the kind my brothers and I grew up on, glued to the TV, twelve inches from the screen when we weren't fighting over the dial on the Magnavox, holding the dial in a death grip, pulling it so hard the TV falls on my arm. That particular family health crisis, unlike so many of Bill's, does not result in a trip to the ER.

The heart failure from which my father had finally expired had been the result of pulmonary pneumonia, but the deep cause of my father's death remains as shrouded in mystery as the nature of his illness while he was alive. That is to say that the immediate cause reveals nothing of the underlying cause(s). The immediate cause just might turn out to be its effect.

My uncle Bob, my father's younger brother and a circuit court judge at the time, presses the VA to change the cause of death to result of a war injury, with all its attendant benefits to the survivors, so we will not sue for negligence. Navy man to the end, Bill had never truly left the service and the service had certainly never left him. He dies on the battlefield of a psych ward at a VA hospital, a prisoner of his own dementia, his death throes tracing inexorably back to 1942. Following in the impossible-for-him-to-fill footsteps of his older brother, Jack—a Seabee who graduated from Notre Dame and Harvard—Bill graduates in English, also from Notre Dame, and enters Midshipmen's School.

While my father was alive I never tried to understand what was the matter with him. I don't think it was because I didn't want to know; I think it was because I didn't think there was anything to find out. I grew up in what I always called a war zone. When you're in the war zone, you don't stop to analyze what's happening, you just try to survive, and then you try to escape.

One of our favorite games was the Great Escape. We turned my brothers' room into a prisoner-of-war camp: two of us are imprisoned in the closet. One plays guard, sitting on the desk with the desk-lamp searchlight. He tries to catch you in the light when you try to make it from the closet over the two twin beds, and through the trench in between, to the wall. If the light catches you, you must return to the closet. If you make it to the wall, you get to be the guard. The trench does double duty: it is also the fort covered with a down comforter, which we call, after my father, the Silly Billy, secured by piles of his old hardcover books that fall on our heads without warning, not unlike his spells. I think of my father as an old green goose-down blanket with multiple scars of holes sewn over, gradually losing his feathers, falling on our heads with the books hard behind. He keeps us warm; he crushes us; we play beneath his darkness.

We called him Little Willy—and used to intone the old nursery rhyme: Little Willy with a shout, gouged the baby's eyeballs out, pounced on him to make him shout, till Mother cried, "William, stop." He would throw his head back and laugh, that marvelous, silky laugh. My mother, with her blue humor, could make him laugh till the tears welled up in his eyes. Little Willy, Silly Billy. After I read *The Hobbit*, I called him Bilbo. They say the number of pet names you have for someone indicates the level of affection.

We watch *Voyage to the Bottom of the Sea*—renamed Voyage to the

Bottom of the Tub because the sub shots are so cheesy—and Efrem Zimbalist Jr. in *The FBI*, one of my father's favorite shows. My brothers and I call it the FBPoop and mock it as hard as we can, but despite the mockery the attraction sticks because later I find I seriously want to join the FBI. Do I want to please my father because *The FBI* is his favorite show? Our other family-favorite show is *Ben Casey*, not surprisingly, in retrospect, about a neurosurgeon. We ridicule the absurdity of the recurrent brain tumors—not grasping the inevitability of that diagnosis on this show—and slam repeatedly through the swinging kitchen door, singing the theme music, as if we're moving into the operating room with tremendous urgency, laughing all the way to cut on somebody's brain AGAIN. My mother devoted her television attention to David Janssen in *The Fugitive*. Maybe because he was always running away or accused of a crime he didn't commit or just because she liked his looks. The film with Harrison Ford so aggravated her that she left the theater in the middle of the show and walked home several miles in the snow. She was seventy-two years old. You get the idea.

I'm five, sitting on my father's lap, pulling the red hair on his chest, which he and I call the Amazon Jungle. We're reading the funny papers and I ask him if he will marry me. He politely declines, explaining to me that he is "already married to your mother." When I disobey my mother, she hits me. When she pulls my pigtails I hold my hair at my scalp so it doesn't hurt, but I act like it's killing me in front of my cousin, who's shocked when I drop the act as soon as my mother leaves the room. I brush it off as if it's nothing. One time my mother reaches for what's handy—the vacuum cleaner cord—but it's always over quickly. My older brother and I devise a sure-fire way to deflect her: at the last moment when she's coming at us we put up all our long bones—shins and forearms—so that she hits her hand on bone and cries, Oh, I broke my hand. Look what you made me do. And it ends there. She never holds grudges, ever, even when she probably has every right to. My father, on the other hand, engages in what he refers to as "psychological warfare": he sends me to my room, his equivalent of solitary confinement. I depend on him to feel guilty fast. I can hear him hovering outside my room: Jo, are you okay? Jo, are you all right? My response is the silent treatment. When he says I can come out, I don't right away because I want to make him feel it. Instead I take out everything he has ever given me, plus the framed photo of his pre-torticollis self in his navy dress uniform that lives on my desk. I hear him give up, his leather slippers—the pair I will keep for years after he is dead and wear sometimes, foolishly amazed that they fit me—shuffling back to the living room. Then I take the stash, sneak out of my room, and shove everything onto my parents' double bed, careful to place his photograph facedown so that he will know what I mean. I betray him back. Two can play at that game.

When he goes and dies ten years later, just as he had told me he would, I apparently still don't know what it means that my father has died. My older brother and I are in his house in Ben Lomond and his friend Andy with the dark Botticelli curls drives me in his beat-up green one-ton Ford truck to the beach so I can see the Pacific for the first time, mysteriously, greenly beautiful in the fog of dawn and I know I've arrived somewhere. When my mother calls us we are in the kitchen of the house and I feel shock—I know my father was sick, but somehow I had no idea that he was dying—and a peculiar, airless relief. Death was the only way out for him. I sound like I'm being reasonable—do I actually speak these ridiculous words or are they only in my head? But I did not anticipate that it would come so early, even though, at the time, it seems too late. I am taken by surprise, because though he's at the VA Hospital, nobody seems to know he might die. I should have known. I could have known. I should have remembered. Didn't he always do what he said he was going to do?

Maybe my version of my father's death is a myth and maybe I'm unwilling to surrender it. In the other version, my father is a desperate man begging for help, who dies alone and abandoned. While he is a patient in the psych ward at Passavant Hospital the year before his death, he chokes on a piece of food—the antipsychotic medication makes it exceedingly difficult for him to swallow—and his heart stops. Technically, he's dead, and something about the other side makes him think that he belongs there. They use the paddles and jolt him back to life. Everybody concurs, including, and most importantly, my father, that they should have let him choke to death, but a hospital can't let him die, at least not that hospital.

Until the early 1990s, care at the VA, in general, was so substandard that Congress considered shutting down the entire system and giving ex-GIs vouchers for treatment at private facilities. The hospitals were dirty, dangerous, and rife with scandals—decomposing bodies of lost soldiers found on the grounds. Maybe my father actually did die on my mother's birthday, but they don't declare him dead until the 26th of August. Maybe there's a cover-up or they simply don't find his dead body for twenty-four hours, in a bed this time instead of on the grounds. He is swallowed up by darkness. My mother never remarries. I've had enough of that, she tells me. I decide that he dies on her birthday in 1975, and she in fact dies on her birthday thirty years after that, their souls bound together to the end.

Doctor Jody

My desire to discover and, more importantly, understand the cause of his decline and death has led me to become something of an armchair neurologist. Sometimes I wish I had become a real neurologist, but in our house, my mother and I shared a profound suspicion of doctors, despite or because of the fact that my mother was a nurse. My father, on the other hand—on the other hand she wore a glove, he would have added, deadpan—had the reverence of a true believer damned by fate. In any event, I declined the six-year medical program at Northwestern because I couldn't stand the thought of touching the bodies of strangers, never considering medical career options that would not have involved touching: like neurology. You can't touch somebody else's brain. Or maybe you can. Maybe I was afraid of finding out what was wrong with my father's brain.

In the sunroom of the house at 620 Wesley Avenue in Oak Park, Illinois, my father is six years old, convalescing from a tonsillectomy. After surgery he suffers a fever, possibly encephalitis contracted during a pandemic of sleeping sickness. It takes him six months to recover. The childhood anesthesia procedure for a tonsillectomy in 1926 is characterized by isolating the child from his mother, wrapping him in a sheet while a nurse attendant forcibly holds the child down to the gurney. A gauze-covered metal cone is clamped over the child's nose and mouth, and ether is dripped from a can onto the gauze while the child screams and thrashes. This procedure alone—without subsequent, possibly brain-scarring, fever—suggests another cause or factor: trauma. By the twenty-first century it is acceptable to consider the neurophysiology of trauma. Robert Scaer, MD, calls spasmodic torticollis an aberration of the orienting reflex, a head twitch worsened by stress and emotion, a response to a perceived threat.

One theory is that Bill caught a virus right after the tonsillectomy, and incurred a brain lesion. A neurologist, who has since died of a brain tumor, once told me that the brain is a house with many rooms, rooms with doors and windows. If a gorilla knocks on the door of one of these rooms, you don't let him in. But if a man who looks like you comes to the door asking for help, you do. When the man asking for help, who is really a gorilla, knocks on the door of six-year-old Bill's brain, Bill lets him in. When it turns out that this gorilla-man has a gun and takes over the room Bill is in, and intends to hold up and take over every other room in his brainhouse, it's too late to stop him. He's in. This gorilla-man is a virus. The fever goes away, but the gorilla-man lies latent in his brain about eighteen years. Then the symptoms start to appear.

I asked my neurologist friend if a brain infection can cause hallucinations, aphasia, psychotic symptoms, paranoia. He said yes, that the windows of the rooms in our brains should stay closed while we're awake, unless we summon particular images as acts of imagination. When we dream, he said, all the doors and windows fly open and flap in the breeze of sleep. A slow virus can eat at the hinges of these doors and windows so that they open involuntarily when you're not sleeping, causing all kinds of horror in my poor father's heart and what was left of his mind, a ruined fresco, a hollow nest for bees.

Me becoming a neurologist just wasn't part of the script. Maybe the hidden script for my life was up in the attic underneath what my mother warned ominously was my father's notoriously, grievously "bad play" called *Strange Music.* I can picture exactly where it was. I never dared or wanted to read it, but one time I did take the lid off the box and something escaped into my world.

The Looney Bin

While I'm an undergraduate at Northwestern, my father is a patient of Dr. Rovner, a neurologist, at Passavant Hospital in downtown Chicago, the Ritz compared to the VA. I take the "L" down to Chicago

Avenue to visit him on weekends. I pick him up at the hospital—he needs a day pass to get out—and we go to Walgreens drugstore on the corner of Chicago and Michigan, order chocolate sodas, and talk about the universe. He is, in these moments, very much himself, or at least whatever I think his self is. Can it be that the order of the ward is what he needs?

"A place for everything and everything in its place." One of his mantras.

Bill is in the psychiatric ward in 1974, his second tour at Passavant Hospital, this time for offenses against his family, at work, and in the street in front of our house. He has an idea that it will be good for him and his family agrees. He knows he's losing control of himself; I think he knows he's losing his mind. I don't know who's responsible for committing him to his first psych ward tour at the VA in 1954—his exile, no doubt, coerced—because my mother is busy at the time, giving birth to me, and Bill is alone, bereft of wife when he wakes up from experimental neurosurgery and threatens to jump out a window. It's probably his neurosurgeon who makes the decision to commit. Mercy Hospital cannot manage a patient with suicidal tendencies, but the VA hospital has to take him. So the neurosurgeon betrays him twice, first by failing in the surgery—and second by committing him to the psych ward at the VA, where he will die twenty-one years later.

Mom (2005): *I should never have allowed that surgery to go on. Well, Bill got some kind of an infection, and so whatever medicine he was taking, maybe phenobarbital for his neck, he had to stop taking it. When I met him he had torticollis, then he's going to M in River Forest and M said to him why don't we do surgery. That's what started it. So we went to who I thought was good, Voris, you know, down at Mercy Hospital. He was a neurosurgeon. He patted Bill's back and said strong back. Poor Bill, you know, after the surgery, and they never shoulda done it, I think now they would have given him an antibiotic or something and it would have worked, I don't think they had it then . . . Maybe the phenobarbital caused the infection.*

Phenobarbital causes the brain to relax. Though my father stops taking phenobarbital, a prescription bottle containing some of the pills lives still in the back of the drawer of my mother's desk in the living room. Brien and I, both toddlers at the time, find it. My mother is napping or simply in another room. When she discovers us with pills in our mouths, she wants to know if we swallowed any. My older brother responds in the negative, but I just smile and laugh, refusing to answer—I must think it's a game—so she has to assume that I might have. Some four hours later, it takes four orderlies to hold me down and by then I am no longer laughing. By the time they get around to actually pumping my stomach, my mother knows, on some nurse level, that had I really swallowed the phenobarbital I would have been unconscious. She believes that this stomach-pumping event changes my personality. Forever after, if I feel backed into a corner I fight back with everything I've got, even if no one is trying to hurt me. My stomach pumping makes the top ten list of things my mother regrets for the rest of her life. Her favorite obsession was to look back at tragedies of the past, particularly grievous parenting errors, and wonder what would have happened if she hadn't done what she'd done. I call it the "if game."

If only she had stopped this procedure from happening, when she knew I couldn't have swallowed any of the drug. If only she hadn't pulled away from the curb like Parnelli Jones—one of our nicknames for her, along with the White Tornado—without knowing my little brother Jack was sitting on the trunk. If she hadn't pulled away so suddenly, then he wouldn't have fallen off the car and hairline-cracked his skull.

Mom (coughing): *See they said Bill was talking about himself right after the surgery. Somebody down at Mercy Hospital said it; I never heard it. That's why they brought him to the VA. He said he'd like to jump out the window or something like that. He wasn't suicidal, he wouldn't. You know he was so Catholic and everything, you know he was so, pardon me, so guilt-ridden, Jesus Christ, about everything. They were crazy, I'm telling you; I'm talking about Grandma. His mother. Guilt, guilt, guilt, guilt, guilt. That's the church, too, at that time. You know Fenwick, Notre Dame, St. Edmunds, the nuns. I remember when there'd be a storm here you know, and I'd tried to be—I didn't want you kids getting goofy about it, and you're not, you weren't. He wanted us to go over to Petersons' basement. From being in the South Pacific in the monsoons.*

In 1961, my father lost his job at U.S. Rubber, where they made Keds. I lived in Keds before I needed corrective shoes, saddle shoes with Thomas heels, for extra bones in my feet: "eminently" (my father's word) mockable clodhoppers. The doctor wanted to do surgery, but my mother wouldn't let him, not after what they did to my father. She was afraid I might never walk again and I was a ballerina. I don't know what Bill did at U.S. Rubber or why he lost his job—my brother says he got laid off from a desk job there because he had to write everything and his hand was shaking: a Parkinsonian symptom resulting from his 1954 surgery. I do remember the day he lost that job, the fear in my mother's eyes, trying to hide a terrible secret that nobody wanted to talk about, hanging in the air like someone died. After he was fired, he sold insurance—his business card says general, auto, fire, life—the desk in the living room stocked with heavy bond stationery perfect for coloring, printed with his name, home address, and the important word Insurance—an irrefutable stack of evidence.

My father always put a high premium on evidence, especially during his "spells." Like a drowning man clutching the shards of an exploded ship, he clung to evidence of the routines of his daily life—plates from breakfast, the clothes he found himself in, the TV guide— to stave off yet another swindling Saturday neurological breakdown. No Sabbath for Bill, despite his faith. He prayed the rosary every night in desperate hope of finding what he sought—peace of mind. That was all he asked for. The Blessed Virgin Mary seemed nonresponsive to him and I couldn't understand why he bothered praying that rosary every night. I thought he was getting rooked. I didn't understand that the act of praying afforded him some small measure of that very peace he was desperately seeking.

He lost his real job—the insurance business was never his real job—at U.S. Rubber and the world got scary for all of us. Big Nurse went back to work on the locked ward and brought home horror stories of her crazy patients. At home, my brothers and I watched *Shock Treatment* and *The Snake Pit*; *One Flew Over the Cuckoo's Nest* comes later, but they're all of a piece—all about people *trapped*, the operative word, in mental wards. These people don't really belong there. I have to ask, did my father?

My recent trip back to *The Snake Pit*, to see if it's half as bad as I remember, proves utterly snake-less, startling me instead with the therapeutic benefits of shock treatment for Olivia de Havilland. Big Nurse in *Cuckoo's Nest* uses shock treatment to punish and control nonconformist McMurphy played by Jack Nicholson, but my father seemed to be a conformist. Maybe life gave him a few shock treatments that knocked him into next week, that made him try to toe the line and play the role of conformist. When I ask my brother if he remembers my father, who claimed to have been an admiral in the Japanese navy, having actual shock treatment, because I think I remember he did, he writes me: "I seem to recall that he was subject to some form of electromagnetic radiation upon his attempted escape from the Japanese Navy in 1943." Who plays Bill in his final scene: Olivia de Havilland or Jack Nicholson? Bill bears a startling resemblance to the gentle, elegant Leslie Howard, star of *Gone with the Wind*, but Leslie is all wrong for this role. I know Bill's not Chief in *Cuckoo's Nest*, smashing through the window, vaulting into the moonlight, flying back into the world free.

I have to think that my father's view of himself changed when he was removed from Mercy and mercy, and committed to the psych ward three days after I was born: his fate was altered. Once you've been committed to a psych ward, you see yourself differently. After the neurosurgery in 1954, he must begin to see himself as somebody who's disintegrating, who's mentally unbalanced, who's failing at being human. If no torticollis—then no surgery. If they could have given him an antibiotic—then they wouldn't have done surgery. If no surgery—no psych ward at the VA and no tremor of the right hand. Twenty years later, he puts looney bin in quotes even as he writes to himself in his diary.

Wednesday 24 April 1974 [first entry]

I'm still in this "looney bin" to try + determine what there is about me that psychologically "ticks" but never as yet quite completely "tocks."

I feel, though, that definite progress has been made in the psychological sector of that most mysterious, selective + indefinable mirage known as the human mind.

For one thing, from the earliest beginning of my life I remember now I was overprotected, was never allowed to accept small responsibilities, which as I grew into manhood, became larger + larger + larger responsibilities, from which my ego, if you want to call it that, recoiled and manifested its dissatisfaction by disintegrating into babyish manifestations such as crying, inability to concentrate, stammering +, in general, evading these responsibilities which had to be faced sooner or later.

Last weekend, though, after having faced the ultimate responsibility of all—twenty years of marriage and three marvelous kids, I recognized the problem. I took the step. I did not try to siphon off the responsibility onto my wife. I planned what we would do and we did it.

I have not worked in a month now and am looking forward to working again. The last weekend at home was a complete uninhibited success. I know what the problem is now. I know how to cope with it. It will not be resolved in a day, a week, or a month. But I do know that I do not need this hospital any more + that periodic visits with Doctor Rovner at his office will suffice. The big thing to remember though, is that I faced this responsibility. I did not try to shirk it or evade it + that today as of these moments I feel like a man and not a baby.

Adios

Mirage in figurative use implies an unrealizable hope or aspiration. He sees the human mind, his, as an unrealizable hope or aspiration, something he'd lost and hoped to find.

He saw his aspiration to become a playwright as a mirage, something quietly surrendered—a manuscript discarded in the attic.

The step to which he refers must have been planning what they would do and doing it. Something banal. Mowing the lawn, going to dinner, going to the movies, going to church, playing Oscar Peterson records, getting through the day, finding something to do tomorrow, getting through the weekend, avoiding a "seizure."

The work he's looking forward to is his occupation as a vocational counselor for the State of Illinois, a real job his brother Bob helped him to obtain after he was fired from U.S. Rubber. His services are provided free of charge to the citizenry. His job description is to help his clients—usually people who have had difficulty finding and holding a job—understand their capabilities and develop career goals. With an awareness of his clients' potential and a knowledge of what skills are in demand in the job market, he provides a link between people looking for work and employers. Somehow this is not a case of the blind leading the blind.

He seems to think that he must heal himself. The neurologist thinks it's purely a matter of Bill's taking responsibility and that it's been such a matter from the very beginning. If this is true, then why is a neurologist even bothering to see Bill?

Time to double the Thorazine.

My brother reminds me that in no appointment with Dr. Rovner was my father ever in one of his full-blown episodes: that is, standing in his track suit on the rug in front of the kitchen door, rocking back and forth from one foot to the other, arms waving up and down, unable to articulate a single word for two hours, hallucinating something having to do with the problem that "the angles are all off," his own vertiginous language evidence of his madness, his body moving in a new way, his mind speaking to itself: "Okay then, all right then, okay then, all right then." The image of a soul in spasm.

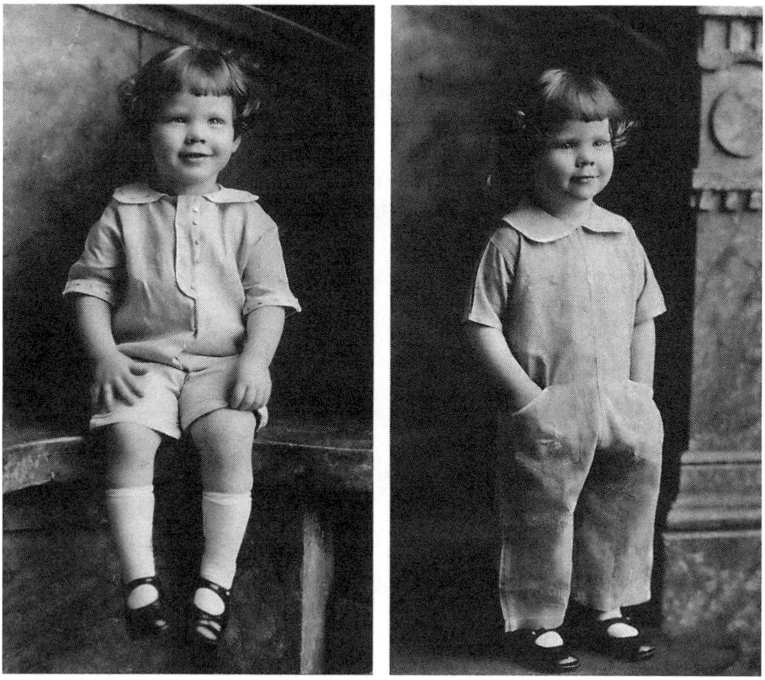

Two faces of Bill as a young child. Everybody thinks these are pictures of Jody.

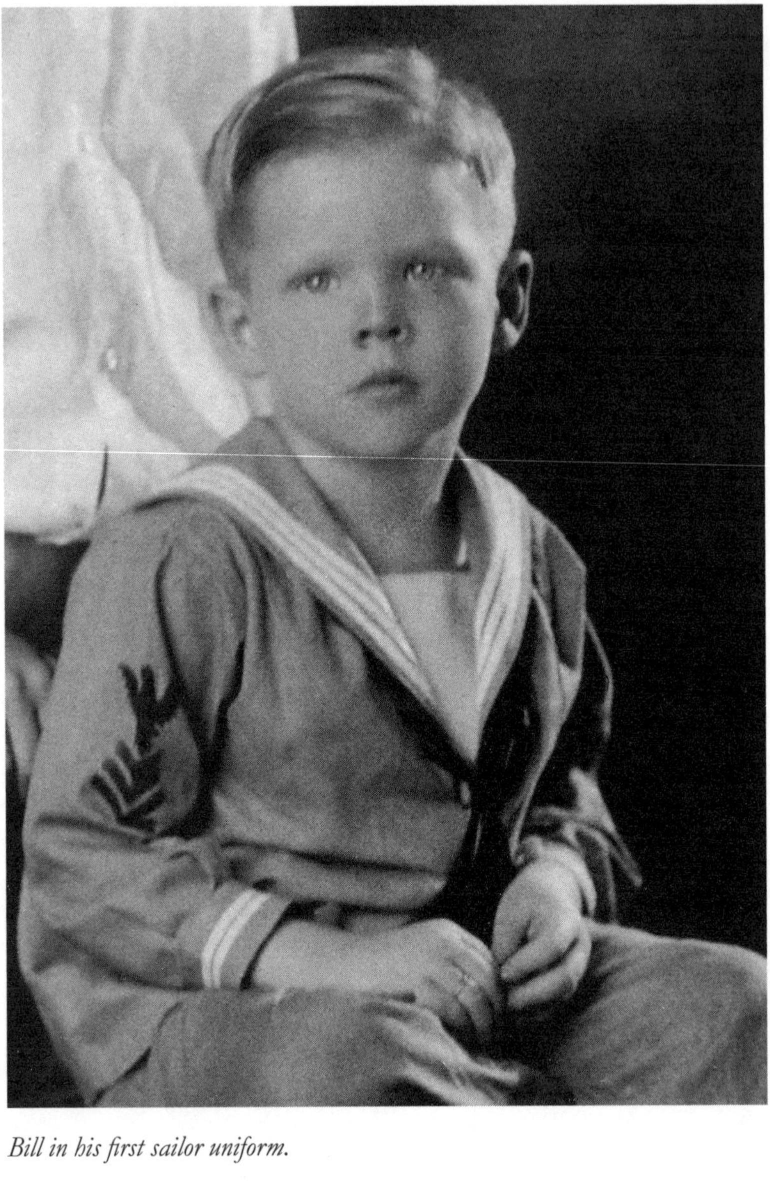

Bill in his first sailor uniform.

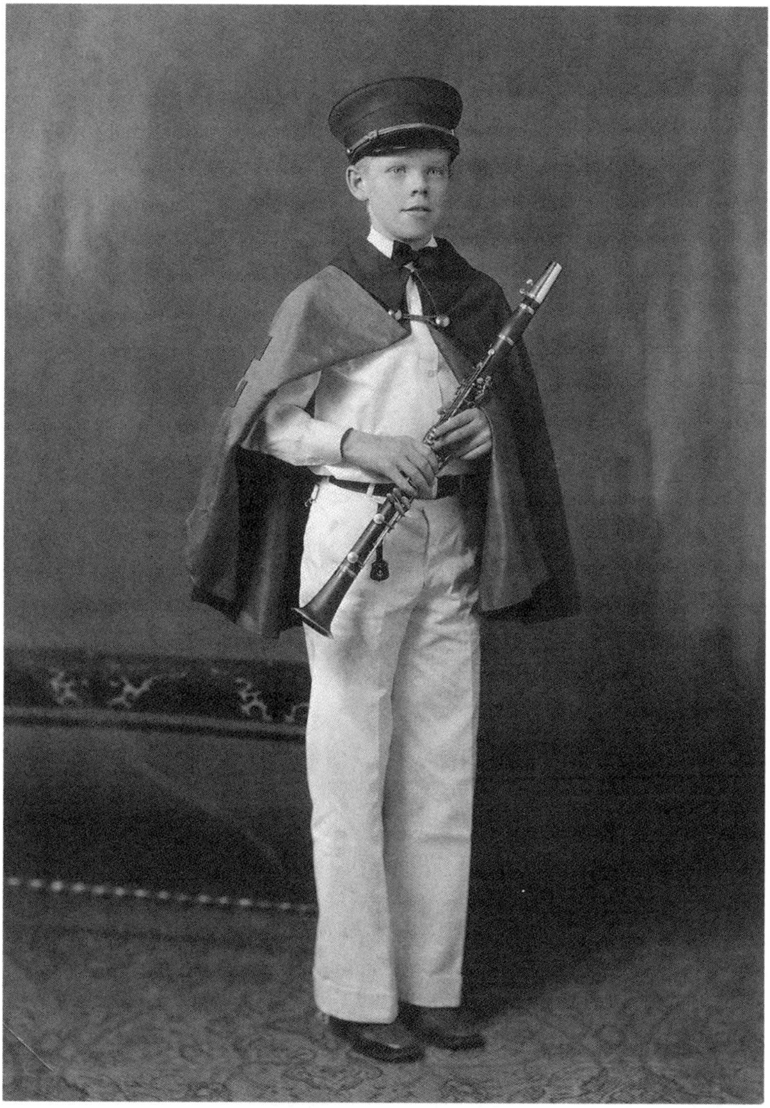

Bill in his band uniform with his clarinet.

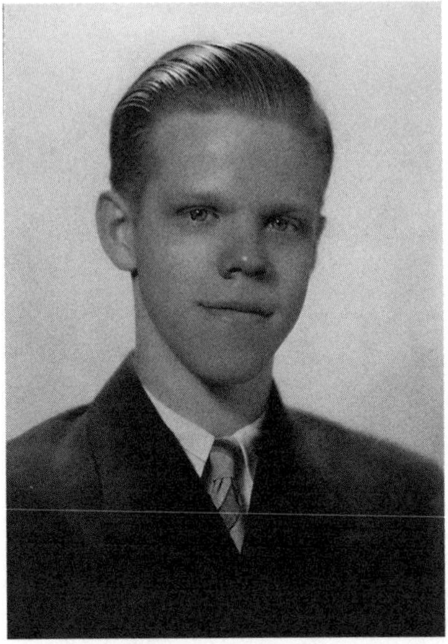

Bill graduates from Fenwick High School, Oak Park, Illinois.

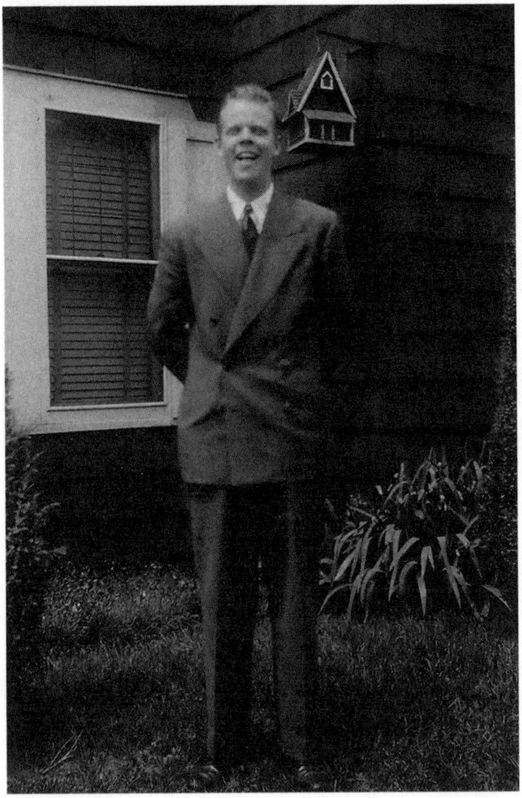

Bill laughing in front of the McAuliffe house on Wesley Avenue in Oak Park.

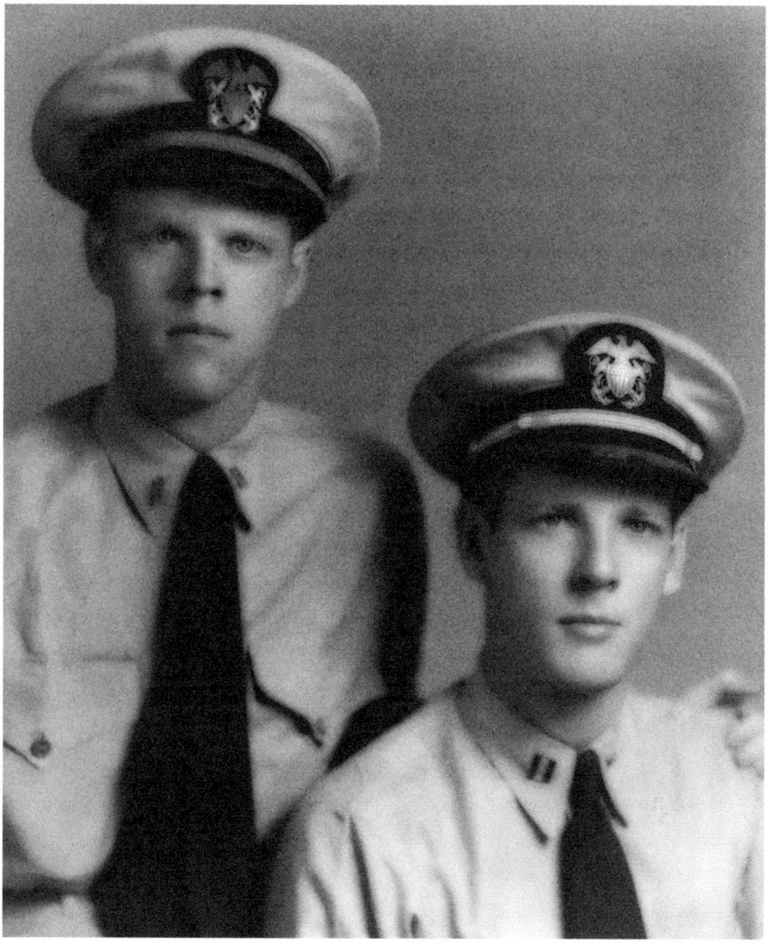

Brother officers in the navy in WWII: Bill on left, and Jack, his older brother.

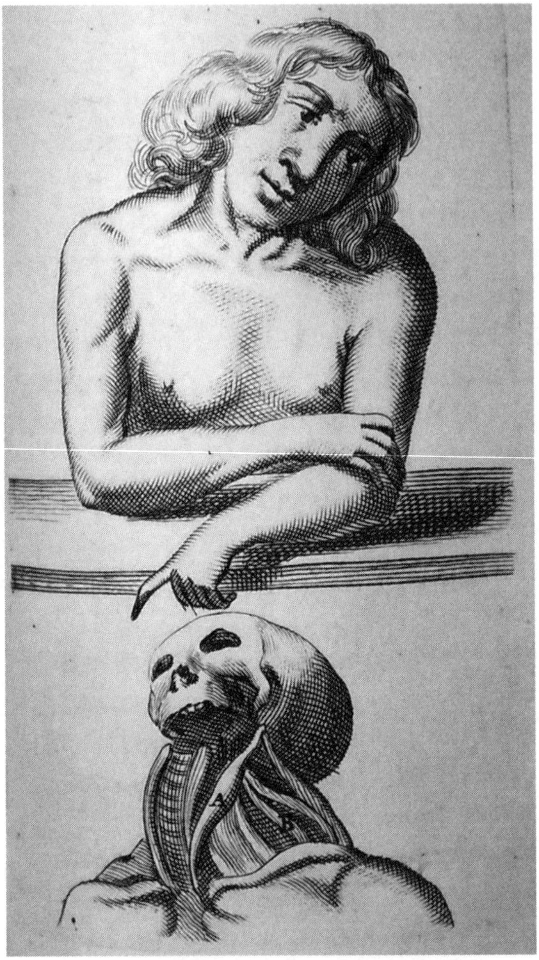

"Pathology of Torticollis," Job van Meek'ren, 1611–1666. Courtesy John Martin Rare Book Room, Hardin Library for Health Sciences, University of Iowa.

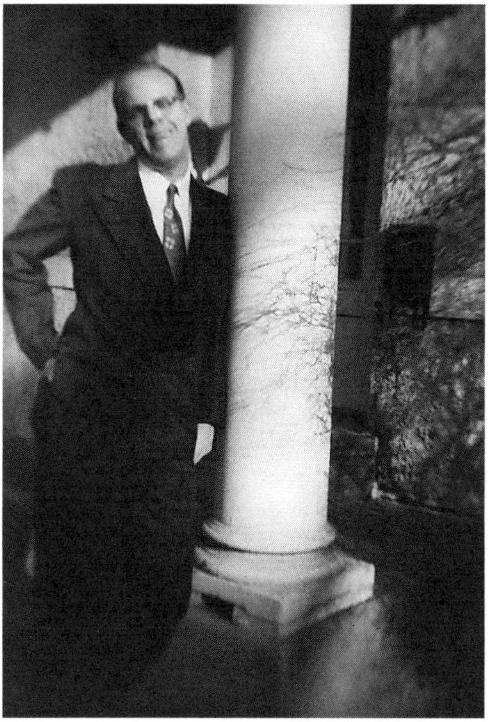

Bill with torticollis, after the war, on Joy's front porch in River Forest, Illinois.

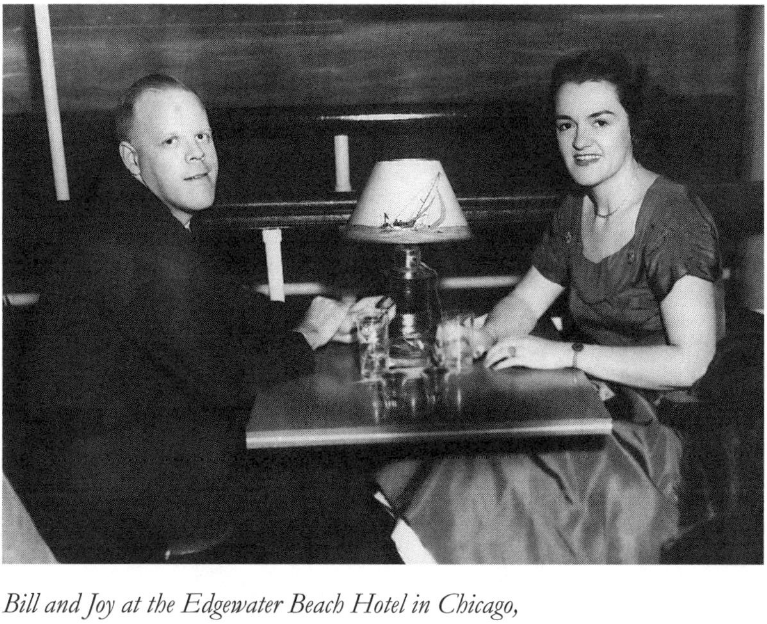

Bill and Joy at the Edgewater Beach Hotel in Chicago, on their honeymoon, January 1953.

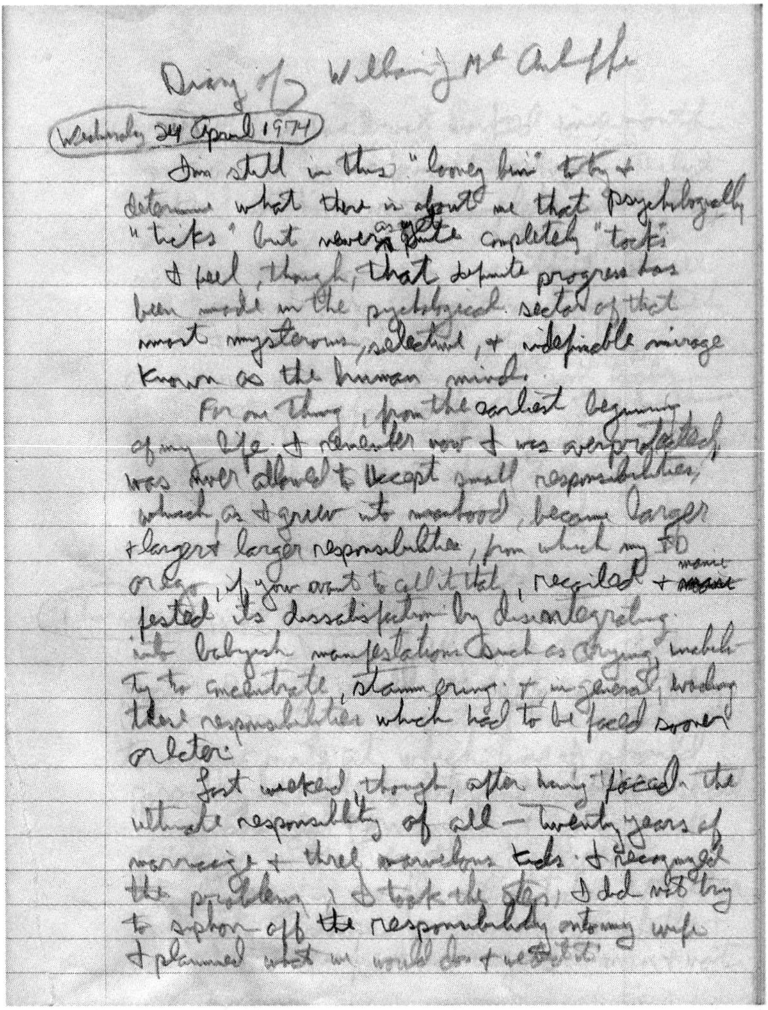
Diary of William J McAuliffe

Wednesday 24 April 1974

I'm still in this "looney bin" to try + determine what there is about me that psychologically "ticks" but never as yet quite completely "tocks".

I feel, though, that definite progress has been made in the psychological sector of that most mysterious, selective, + indefinable mirage known as the human mind.

For one thing, from the earliest beginning of my life I remember now I was overprotected, was never allowed to accept small responsibilities, which as I grew into manhood, became larger + larger + larger responsibilities, from which my ID or ego, if you want to call it that, recoiled + manifested its dissatisfaction by disintegrating into babyish manifestations such as crying, inability to concentrate, stammering, + in general, avoiding those responsibilities which had to be faced sooner or later.

Last weekend, though, after having faced the ultimate responsibility of all — twenty years of marriage + three marvelous kids. I recognized the problem, I took the step, I did not try to siphon off the responsibility onto my wife I planned what we would do + we did it.

First page of my father's diary, begun during his stay at Passavant Hospital in Chicago, dated April 24, 1974.

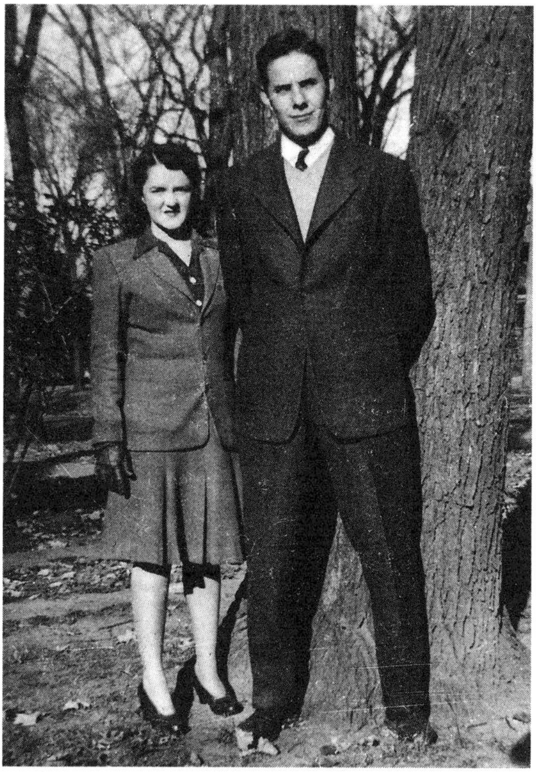

My mother in River Forest, Illinois, with her fiancé, Ralph, who was lost in WWII.

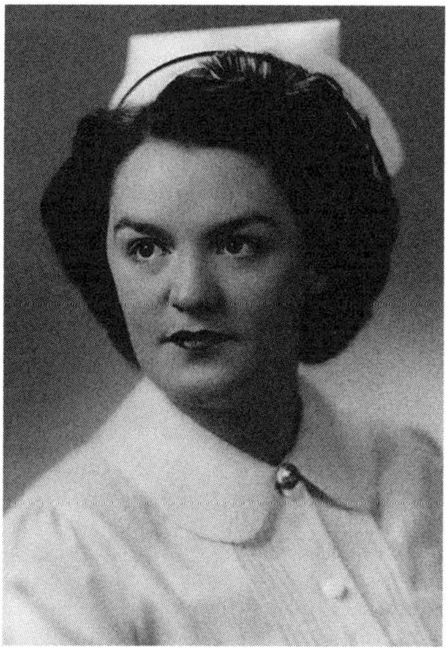

Mercedes J. O'Brien graduates in the class of 1947 from St. Anne's Hospital School of Nursing in Chicago.

Part Two

Far safer, of a Midnight Meeting
External Ghost
Than its interior Confronting—
That Cooler Host.

C. 1863, EMILY DICKINSON

Little Willy

William (Bill) Joseph McAuliffe—Mc + Olaf, redheaded Viking ought-to-be—is born on November 14, 1920, the third of four children of John H. McAuliffe and Margaret Cronin. As an infant, so the story went, my grandmother lived in a cabin in Montana surrounded by "Indians." She was born in the Nez Percé Indian lands in Bitterroot Valley in 1892 and is believed to have been the first white child born in Montana. Flo Ziegfeld asked this former novitiate nun, convent dropout, to go to New York and be in the Follies, but she declined, the path too far from her convent upbringing. These last details bear an uncanny resemblance to the life of Mary Tyrone, the mother in Eugene O'Neill's autobiographical tragedy, *Long Day's Journey into Night*, with the notable exception that my grandmother was not addicted to morphine, even if she did like her Old Fashioned.

Old Fashioned for her, Shirley Temple for me, and she always lets me eat her maraschino cherries.

Whenever she takes me and my two girl cousins out to one of her special, girls-only lunches at places sounding like plantations—the Homestead or Lawn Grove—she leaves my older brother standing on the curb waving bye-bye as she pulls away in her big green Buick, the leather seats smelling of her rose perfume. Happy to be a member of the club, I'm too dumb to say, I want my brother to come, too.

Let's face it: the real Mary Tyrone in my outfit is indubitably (his word) my father, the one who holds us all in a thrall of terror that he will flip out, lost to the haze of the past or the abyss of the future. It's the pain of childbirth and a vagabond existence made up of cheap doctors and homelessness that condemn Mary Tyrone to harrowing drug addiction and madness. Grief, loss, and Irish weakness for addiction entrench the syndrome. No bleating foghorn for us as in O'Neill's play, just the intermittent watch/warning of tornado trailing ominously across the bottom of our TV screen. *Long Day's Journey* is the first play I work on when I start directing in my first year of graduate school.

Margaret Cronin, my father's mother, grew up a religious fanatic and brilliant card player who religiously had her nails done once a week, even as she lay, for ten years, with the left side of her body paralyzed from a stroke that followed hard upon the news of my father's early death at fifty-four, her visceral reaction evidence of their emotional connection. When private care for Bill became too expensive for my parents to bear, Grandma—in deep denial of what was really the matter with my father and apparently, says my brother, locked in a mutual blamefest with my mother—refused to help. My grandfather had left her very well taken care of when he passed away in 1955. She was in Hawaii visiting her eldest son in the summer of 1975 when she heard that Bill was lost, this time forever. Post stroke, Grandma had no interest in rehabilitation.

Big Jack

My younger brother, Jack (2009): *As I started to get through high school the whole home situation became much worse, and then it was just basically chaos all the time on weekends and you just lived in fear of the next episode, and he deteriorated further into very little time in between episodes, if any, and then when I was a junior, Mom had him committed to Hines. He was in Passavant for a certain amount of time but they couldn't afford it so they put him in Hines. Grandma wasn't on board and she certainly wasn't on board with Hines. She was outraged. They didn't know that anything was happening. It was like when* [Aunt] *Mary and* [Uncle] *George were sitting there at the kitchen table and I was describing the scene when he was running around outside in his underwear, and I was embarrassed, ashamed, and they both started in on me, they started yelling at me about How would you react if he had a heart ailment would you be ashamed of that?! You know it's the same thing! And Mom just stood by and there was no one there to defend me. There was no one to defend me ever. And by the time he went into Hines he basically just checked out and was ready to go. Again after he died, they had a meeting at the house to figure out what they were going to do about this thing and I said, well he wanted to die anyway, and they all started yelling at me about that, too. So I get that just after my father died. Bob and Mary and again, no one defended. No one. They shoulda sent me away.*

I remember when Jack was four: he had to be at least four because he was riding a bicycle, the Schwinn. I wanted to go to Aunt Betty's, Uncle Bob's wife, and what did Jack do? He took off on his bike to go over to get Brien, who was behind where the police station is now on Roosevelt Road. Mother didn't know where he went. She took me to Betty's and she was going to come back and get Jack. In the meantime Jack saw her going to Betty's and he followed on his bike. He got to 25th Avenue and he was trying to cross the street, a *little* guy, and some truck driver stopped and got him across the street. He made it to Betty's, and I said to him: Momma was just here, you go home. When she came back over to me, I said, I sent him back. Oh Jesus Mercy, said my mother. So she went down the street after him. He had gone down 24th to try and get across there. That's where she got him. He was crying; he was afraid. He knew crossing 25th was hard, beyond him.

There are so many things wrong with this picture that it's too easy to find them. Seven years old, supposedly the age of reason, I send him back. Fear of my mother made me send my four-year-old brother back across such a busy street. I did not defend him. They should have sent Jack to Hawaii, the place, in my family, where dreams are born or broken.

Here Be Dragons

My grandmother, Dad's mom, gives me a book about Hawaii when I am a little girl. In 1967, my older brother, thirteen, spends the summer in Kailua, gets stung by a jellyfish and contracts walking pneumonia. He never goes back. I finally make it there in 1985, only to discover, at long last, what I thought was the most beautiful place on earth, as close to heaven as it's possible to ascend, the mountain tops wearing the clouds like garlands in their black wavy hair in the mornings after the rains. I play the piano on the lanai in the off hours in the house that Uncle Jack built and Aunt Mary Jane tells me how much I put her in mind of my grandfather. She says it's like having him back in the house again. The idea of being my grandfather's ghost fits me like my father's old slippers.

My grandfather, Dad's father, a fantastic jazz pianist, inherits his father's musical talent, and puts himself through law school in Chicago playing nights in what were then called "saloons," unfettered by the perfectionist restrictions that will severely limit my father's artistic aspirations. The first McAuliffe to graduate from Notre Dame, precocious Grandpa passes the Bar at age twenty, but can't practice law until his twenty-first birthday. A lawyer's lawyer and noted trial attorney, he owns a five-bedroom cottage on the beach in Long Beach, Michigan. Their life a picture of moneyed success, my grandparents name both the cottage and their boat Marymac after their first child and only girl, Mary, on whom the sun rises and sets. The sun only sets on my father.

During the limo ride to my father's burial in Queen of Heaven Cemetery, Bob, who had worked in my grandfather's law office, leans his basset hound face toward me meaningfully and asks if I ever wondered how my father's family had managed to live so well during the Depression. He suggests that my grandfather—whose neighbors in Long Beach included Tony "Big Tuna" Accardo, Paul "the Waiter" Rica, and Lucky Luciano—had business dealings with the Mafia. Sally S, the young girl next door in Michigan City, who came to love my father when he stayed with her family after the war, denies my grandfather's involvement in any such activity, but how could she, a nine-year-old, have known? Her mother, a corporate client of my grandfather's, considered him "next to God."

During that infamous (one of my father's words) ride to the cemetery, Bob also takes the opportunity to tell me with characteristic offhanded bitterness that my grandmother and Aunt Josie, her aunt, overprotected my father when he was a child. According to my mother, Bill "couldn't hold a hammer."

Bob does not comment on the fact that he and my father's older sister, Mary, scrupulously carried on that tradition of overprotection by jumping on any threat to Bill, which usually translated to jumping on my little brother. Maybe my father needed protection, or gave the impression that he did, after recuperating for six months from the post-tonsillectomy infection. Not allowed to do for himself, he becomes somebody who must rely on the protection of others. Why—or if—Bill becomes constitutionally incapable of accepting larger responsibilities is not clear. Perhaps his adult neurological disorder is tied to his particular personality type as, for example, sufferers of essential tremor tend to be very detail-oriented, wrapped tighter than the rest of us. In the 1920s, torticollis was considered regression to an infantile type of habit; its tenderminded, sensitive sufferers were thought to have trouble with superiors, and feelings of inferiority and self-pity. It may be true that he was never allowed to accept small responsibilities, but his memories of this could be so-called "recovered," evidence planted by his neurologist, who, my brother kindly says, was working with the tools available to him at the time, what seem to me barbaric tools of blame and guilt.

Is torticollis a neuropsychiatric disease, entailing cognitive changes that sometimes progress to dementia? My neurologist friend says no. I seem to remember my mother telling me that during an autopsy they discovered that my father had brain lesions—or was it scar tissue in the grey matter? My brother does not recall any autopsy, but the death certificate says there was one. Stress made Bill's symptoms worse and my mother was a stress machine for him, just as he was for her. The two together generated a perfect storm of stress. "Just checking," he repeats the obsessive-compulsive mantra, hopelessly sandbagging, arranging objects on his bureau, trying to hold it together against the inevitable Saturday storm. It's as if his navy uniform were permanently rotting off his body, the living room a veritable monsoon trough, as he spins on the rug in the kitchen door: monsoon internalized. Bill seems lost in what he described as that most "mysterious, selective + indefinable mirage known as the human mind," unaware that at least half of him is actually ruled by creatures lurking in that unmapped zone of his brain—the part labeled "here be dragons."

The family history tells of art, specifically music, as the engine for success—not an end in itself, but the means to an end. This formula never jells for my father, erstwhile clarinetist, or his older sister Mary, so-called concert pianist. Bob and Jack can't be bothered with studying music; they're headed for professional school. My mother once told me that of the McAuliffe boys, she got the best one. Uncle Jack, key figure in building the airfield from which the B-29 *Enola Gay* took off in order to drop the atomic bomb on Hiroshima, fits the family profile to a T: handsome officer (rear admiral in the reserve), thorough gentleman, successful architect, fine golfer. After the war, he decides to stay in Hawaii—as far away from his mother as he can get. Neither the navy nor Hawaii agrees with my father. His mother remains inescapable.

Bob, drafted into the army in WWII straight out of high school, becomes a prison guard for prisoners of war in Georgia. After the war he returns to Oak Park and attends the University of Chicago, where he lives down the hall from a future serial murderer who scrawls in lipstick on the bathroom mirror: Please stop me. Mary's army sergeant husband's posting to Japan after the war gives her a new life in a magical world: Japan defines her taste, shapes her movements, and alters her identity, but not enough to keep her from returning to a tiny apartment on Maple Avenue in Oak Park, just a few blocks from her mother.

When Bill was born, my grandparents were living at the Oak Park Arms, a luxury hotel with a ballroom, which my grandfather had at one time owned. Hemingway hailed from Oak Park, too. Older than my father by twenty-one years, he had grown up down the street from the apartment on Oak Park Avenue, where my widowed grandmother died half-paralyzed, having exhausted her fortune on round-the-clock nurse's aides. Oak Park—which Hemingway referred to as a town "with wide lawns and narrow minds"—is next door to River Forest, where Frank Lloyd Wright built his house on the rustic corner of Forest and Chicago avenues, my mother's house around the corner. Hemingway went to the same high school as my mother, but my father and his brothers all went to Fenwick, the all-boys Catholic high school in Oak Park. Hemingway's future was mapped out for him: writing, depression, shock treatment, loss of memory, inability to work, paranoia, a shotgun to the head. If my father, whose deepest talent was writing, hadn't been such a devoted Catholic, he may have considered a shotgun as his final exit. Hemingway knew that the river beyond the cedar ahead went into the swamp, where the fishing is tragic. The creatures who live there have to stay low to the ground to live at all. No crashing. No walking. Reading is better, that is if you have something to read. The future is an impossible place, water up to your armpits and no sun. Hemingway's hero, Nick Adams, the opposite of articulate Bill, can go back to camp: he can fish the swamp later. But once the gorilla with the gun is in Bill's head, fishing the swamp becomes an inevitability.

Thursday April 25, 1974 [second entry]

I had fully expected that Doctor Rovner would be over to see me today but apparently he is out of town until tomorrow nite at which time I should possibly be able to determine whether I shall be discharged permanently and go to work Monday or not. Everything apparently hinges on my performance today. Whether I start stammering and stuttering or whether I can still keep functioning as a man and not a little baby. Anyway last night we took a trip to the Art Institute which was very enjoyable + I still did feel a little withdrawn, conversationally speaking. However, I am making a constant effort to capitalize on small talk + conversation on a social level. This, I am sure, I can + will do.

Adios

His disintegrations bear no resemblance to any babyish behavior I have ever seen. In a man with such a highly developed vocabulary, my father's concern about stammering and stuttering and withdrawal, "conversationally speaking," are red flags.

Brother Jack (2009): *You didn't talk about battle fatigue, it was shameful. You know about George Patton slapping a soldier. Well it's a bad public relations thing but it's certainly a feeling: if everybody had battle fatigue you'd lose the war. If it were everybody on both sides, then the war would stop. We tried that in WWI where everybody stopped for awhile and they were going to kill them. Their officers were going to kill them if they didn't get back in the trenches. You have to have order in the ranks; it's fundamental to military thinking.*

Rebel with a Cause

My mother tells me Bill had flaming red hair just like mine when I was born, but I can't believe it because, in real life, his hair looks blonde. Mine is blonde now, too. The process starts at twenty-five:

that's when the color starts to fade. That's just after he got torticollis. She shows me the pictures and he looks exactly like me, which makes me feel good because I want to look like my father. I don't want to look like my mother. I look like him and then I know who I am and how things are with me, where I come from, what I'm like. He's smiling and sitting on a stone bench with his hair curled and wearing short bangs—he looks like a girl, or maybe it's the style of the time, or maybe it isn't and he has a striking feminine aspect. In another picture, it must have been the same day because his hair and the setting are so similar, he wears a jumpsuit and his hands are in his pockets—he looks like a little man, relaxed and full of purpose. In another when he may have been six, he wears a sailor suit, navy-cursed from the get-go, and a tiny gold ring on his right hand. His hair parted and combed, he looks already like someone with a highly developed interior life, all curves and tucked under himself, but not yet writhing and contorted. Then the school picture from 1927 when he was seven, lips pursed into a grin, and he looks positively impish, even with his hands carefully folded one over the other before an open book. Carrot top. Snake in the grass.

When the McAuliffes move into the house on Wesley Avenue, Aunt Josie comes to help my grandmother with the children. My grandfather complains that she came for three weeks and stayed for thirty years. A religious fanatic like my grandmother, she is forever repeating herself and always talking weather. The house bursting at the seams, my grandfather retreats to the second floor like Ibsen's *John Gabriel Borkman*—except my grandfather, John Herbert, chooses his isolation. Scandal—a fraud Borkman committed—imposes isolation on him: he's the wolf at the top of the stairs, whose footfalls haunt his wife and sister-in-law, both his former intimates, beneath him. Both men take their meals alone. Does my grandfather take his meals privately to get away from his wife and her aunt, or is it simply due to the gout: after a hard day's work he can't bring himself to walk down and up the stairs again. Gout prevents him making any sounds of footfalls. Does he make any sound at all? Does he haunt those below? There was sure never anything going on between Josie and Grandfather. Do Grandma and Josie struggle to get young Bill for themselves? Are we talking melodrama or farce?

The first play my father writes in high school is entitled *6:30 at*

620—about the dinner hour at the house. Every Friday night my grandparents dress formally and head to the club for bridge and dancing. Bridge is serious business for the McAuliffe clan. Dinner hour at our house was a theatrical event: no phone calls allowed. My father's sensibility about language and behavior is strictly heightened: if we say "she," referring to our mother, he says, Who is "she"? Your mother is not "she." If I don't want to eat something green, he counters, You love it, you love it, you love it. The kitchen table was an opportunity for a scene. At Saturday morning breakfast, he'd say Let's talk about the universe. That was before Saturday sucked the universe into a black hole.

Bill and his sister Mary seem to inherit the musical talent from their father, but the first thing Bill does when he returns from the war—he sells his clarinet. He doesn't need the money. He needs to cut himself off. He needs to close that door. I always wondered how he could have done such a thing—betrayed himself in that way, but now it seems painfully obvious: how can you play the clarinet when your head jerks uncontrollably to one side? He never gives torticollis as a reason for why he stopped playing clarinet. His explanation to me was that he could never improvise like Benny Goodman, this despite his awareness that Benny Goodman's solos were written out. Only a member of a family of overachievers could come up with a reason like that. Survivors. Artistic self-starters. My father does not fit the profile. Bill's sister, the concert pianist who takes the pseudo-Russian Marya as a professional name, wasn't good enough, according to Bill. Does the perfectionism come from within or without, something he contracts like a virus from the very atmosphere at 620 South Wesley Avenue, borne down the stairs from the highly successful, gout-afflicted father? Maybe Bill's brain is already misfiring, the darkness having already begun to set in. Nine months before his death, in a prescribed search for a sideline he can enjoy doing, he will return, at everybody's insistence, to his old friend and nemesis the clarinet. He will try, but it will be too difficult. He will not know all the sharps and flats. He will have forgotten some of the fingerings.

Or . . .

He never wanted to play the clarinet and only did it because it was expected of him. He didn't like doing it. He never wanted to be a musician. First chance he gets, he sells his clarinet. It's not a tragedy, it's a liberation. The rebel against the family inheritance wants to be a writer. Nine months before he dies, he will use writing in an attempt to reconcile the insuperable deluge of depression and despair that he will be feeling. As far as doing things that he will like to do, he will be writing, writing to overcome some of his feelings when he is home again from the hospital.

In the band photo, maybe he is twelve, he looks breakable inside the perfect uniform, the band cape cast in perfect jauntiness over his right shoulder, his fingers delicately touching his clarinet, crisp white shirt and cuffed pants, a bow tie and a military cap, his fragile eyes, his lips just slightly parted on the verge of acquiescence. He whispers: I would rather be writing. The uniform looks too heavy for his slender glass frame. Who's making him play that thing—his mother? His father's at work or upstairs with his foot off the ground. I get a taste of Bill's rigorous aesthetic when he wants me to choose, at the age of nine, my own artistic fate. He poses the question: Do you want to be in the circus (his own translation of gymnastics) or the ballet? I know what the right answer is and I give it to him. I suppose I could have chosen the circus, but there's something in the way he frames the question that makes it eminently clear that ballet is better. After I dance with the Kirov and in *The Nutcracker* in Chicago, Marya gets me an in with Walter Camryn, whom she knew in her brief professional career. Walter and his partner Bentley Stone run the best ballet school in Chicago. I'm so young I don't understand that I can leave my ballet body behind at the studio. I try too hard, even then, smiling hard enough to break my face. I take that ballet body, the forced turnout and the bleeding toes, the cracked smile, and wear it all the time like a hand-me-down suit two sizes too small, locking my ribcage—the better to protect my heart—and locking my pelvis—the better to crush the colon that will require surgery (laparoscopic resection) when I'm fifty. Always nothing if not a good student, I'm holding it all together, just like Dad.

At ten years old I take the subway downtown from Des Plaines, the same one my dad takes every day to work. Well past the time I am twelve—I'm pretty short at that age so I can mostly get away with it—my mother makes me lie and say I'm under twelve so that I only have to pay twelve cents to ride to Madison and Wells, where Stone-Camryn sits a few doors down from the "L" tracks. I hate having to lie. Sometimes the lady in the change booth presses me—she can't believe I'm eleven when I'm actually anywhere from twelve to fifteen—she makes me sweat, but I persevere, insisting that I'm only eleven. I don't want to disappoint my mother. She survived the Depression. I know the value of a nickel. My grandmother warns me that someone might try to shoot me full of heroin and kidnap me, and worries why I don't have my period yet, hounding my mother about it till the doctor puts me on thyroid pills. When anybody on the train looks at me cross-eyed, I pretend to be both spastic *and* mental, because I think one of these bizarre behaviors couldn't possibly be enough to keep potential marauders at bay. I do have my reasons for thinking somebody might want to kill me. Once an old man offers me a piece of candy, and my head practically explodes. I think it's D-Day. I back away from him and he stops.

Near the end, Bentley says to Walter—not to me though I am standing right there because dancers are like racehorses—I think she will dance. This is the seal of approval, the signal that you must go to New York when you're eighteen. When Walter asks me if it's hard for my family to pay for ballet lessons, I'm so embarrassed that I say no, even though it is hard on my father's civil servant's salary. I don't understand that he's trying to put me on scholarship. Shame blinds me to the salvation of his subtext. When I decide to quit ballet at sixteen, it seems all or nothing to me, just like the clarinet to my father. New York at eighteen or bust: plan B, quit ballet and go to college. Stop dancing forever. Improvise like Benny Goodman or sell your clarinet. This time when I have to choose, I choose college. My brain needs to feed. She won't dance after all.

November 7, 1972

Dear Jody,
You were right; it was kind of a raunchy Saturday for me, but, fortunately I recovered sufficiently to go to work yesterday. Today being election day + a holiday for me, Joy + I seen our duty + we done it; in other words, we voted. I voted the straight Communist ticket + Joy voted for the more conventional candidates. Seriously, though, I hope McGovern wins, although I don't think he has much chance.

I'm off Friday too for Veterans' Day so I'm sure getting my share of holidays this month. That's what I would like most of all: a work month where the holidays outnumbered the working days, but such a situation would be too ghastly to even think of.

I just wanted to let you know that I really enjoyed getting your letter; it cheered me up immensely.

Hope your play is coming along well + I know that you'll be a big success in it. I firmly believe that your true vocation is the theatre and that you have a great talent for it.

I'm taking the 14th off too because it's my birthday. Take care of yourself, honey

Love,
Dad

Nothing to Be Done

My mother's eighty-fourth birthday, the day she decides to die, comes on August 24, 2005. My mother has to die before I can write about my father. Sally, my mother's hospice nurse, calls me on Tuesday, August 22nd. She says that my mother is not doing well and has taken a very bad turn. She had, in fact, stopped eating on the Saturday before. Sally knew only that she hadn't eaten Monday or Tuesday because Dorota (Dorothy), Mom's caregiver, had been away that weekend. Sally said that once a person with idiopathic pulmonary fibrosis stops eating, they don't last the week. I asked her how long she thought she'd last and she said she didn't know, couldn't say. Sally said she thought I'd better come. I asked her to give the phone to my mother. She did. I said Hi and Mom said, I'm not dead yet. I had only to decide if I would go that day, Tuesday, or Wednesday morning. I talked to my brother Jack after Sally called him. He said if I wanted to be there for him, Wednesday was fine, but if I wanted to be there for Mom it would have to be today. I told my husband I had to go, made a reservation, and helped him pack the two FedEx boxes for Italy. My husband, daughter, and I were going to Florence for the fall semester. My mother knew I was due to leave on Sunday. He drove me to the airport. I took all my Italy stuff not knowing when I would leave or where I'd be going. I got to Chicago in the evening and called from the car to have Dorothy tell my mother I was coming, that I'd be there shortly. I wanted her to know.

When I arrived at the house Mom was in bed. I came in to see her and she said, I'm glad you're here. She was bone thin. Dorothy and I helped her sit on the commode. Getting her off of it and back into bed was awkward for us—like trying to maneuver long sticks. I felt bad because I wasn't able to do it well, make it comfortable for my mother. But we did the best we could and I tried to straighten her out and fix her pajamas once she was back in the bed. We went to sleep to the familiar sound of the oxygen machine pumping away. She had refused the oxygen from Dorothy once that evening but then Dorothy got her to take it.

When I got up in the night to pee I went in to check on Mom and she was lying on her side facing the window, breathing. I went back to bed. When I woke up the next morning I heard Dorothy and Mom arguing, it sounded like, and Dorothy knocked on my door and asked me to come. I came at once. Dorothy said she won't take the oxygen and I said to put it where she can reach it if she wants it. Mom was still lying on her side. Dorothy set the tube near her hand. Joy pushed it away with a strong, fierce move and said, I don't want it! I said that we couldn't force her. I didn't know how long she would live without oxygen from the machine. I went to the right side of the bed, my dad's side, and sat down. I said to Dorothy, You better call Jack, and she did. It was five to seven. Mom lay on her back. She held my left hand tightly and I held hers back. She said, I'm dying, and I said, I know and I love you so much. She said, Let me go. Dorothy came back and said that Jack would be there in five minutes. Mom was looking up and she breathed with labor periodically. Jack arrived and sat on the bed. Mom said, Off bed. I said I thought it was because it made her feel as if the bed were tilting or uneven. Jack stood up. I said to stand where she could see him. He did. I said, Jack's here Mom, and he said, I'm here Mom. I sat there suspended not knowing if she were dead or alive, not sure if she would breathe again and not sure exactly when she left us. The breath came as a surprise—a gasp—and then nothing until finally she didn't breathe anymore. I sat with her there like that for awhile, there in the room where we had talked so many times over fifty years, the room that was always open to me, my parents' bedroom next door to my room, next door to my brothers' room. I thought how dignified her death was, how fitting for her to die in her own bed, to control the circumstances the way she did, to have nothing stuck in her. She had asked for water at one point and Dorothy tried to give it to her but she couldn't swallow. She was brave when she faced it, looking up with such courage and calm.

I didn't cover her up with the sheet. I fixed her pajamas and touched her face. I guess I thought she should stay just as she was. Even after we left the room I came back to look at her. The hospice nurse arrived at 9:15 and declared her dead. She pulled the sheet to cover her body.

I fly to Italy the day after the funeral so I'm not there when my brother and my cousin clean out the house. That playscript of Bill's, *Strange Music*, sitting for half a century in the attic to the right of the stairs until my mother dies, disappears into thin air. Now I can never read the play, but I can hear the music floating down through the eaves like fine dust.

Part Three

Far safer, through an Abbey gallop,
The Stones a'chase—
Than Unarmed, one's a'self encounter—
In lonesome Place—

C. 1863, EMILY DICKINSON

Beach Boss

Sometime after my mother dies, my brother finds Dad's obituary in the *Oak Leaves* among my mother's papers.

> 9/24/75. A long time resident of Oak Park, William J. McAuliffe, 54, died August 26, 1975 after a long illness. Mr. McAuliffe, son of the late John H. McAuliffe and Margaret, came to OP when he was 8 months old and spent his early years at the family home at 620 Wesley Ave. He attended St. Edmund School and Fenwick HS where he was graduated with honors. After receiving a degree from Notre Dame University, he was commissioned an ensign in the Navy in 1942. He served 3 years on an LST in the South Pacific, serving as 'beach master' during assaults on the Gilbert Islands. He took part in some of the worst engagements of the war, including the assault on Saipan and other Pacific Islands. Upon returning from service, he entered the University of Hawaii for graduate studies in English and the theater. Later he came back to OP to live and was active in the St. Edmund Players, while also engaging in the business.

This sterling tale of heroism in the South Pacific does not jibe with what my brother had heard from my father's younger brother, Bob. Jack sends to the U.S. Navy for documents relating to my father's participation in WWII. The documents that he receives in return do not tell the whole story. He has to parse the Notice of Separation from the U.S. Naval Service and the Statement of Service for me. My father sure wasn't talking. Bill was on active duty in the South Pacific for a year and a month from January 1943 to February 1944. He gave Student as his last employer, having graduated from Notre Dame with a major in English in May of 1942, member of the glee club and fencing team.

We conclude the obit must have been written by his sister Mary, with her lifelong penchant for fantasy. Bill was a beach boss, but he didn't make it past a year and a month. His personal island-hopping didn't extend beyond the Gilbert Islands. Contrary to the impression my aunt was trying to make, my father was not a war hero in the traditional sense.

Beach boss is slang for beachmaster of a landing craft. An artillery spotter for the Marines, he coordinates troops on the beaches and communicates with the ships at sea, using signal flags, blinker lights, and radios. He has to stay on the beach a long time; he's supposed to stay cool under pressure. He's been doing this assignment for more than six months. He's supposed to get promoted after six months because it's wartime, but his commanding officer doesn't promote him—because he hates him, because Bill's failing, or both. On night watch he thinks he sees something. Was it just that he was afraid? He wakes the captain up, but there's nothing, and does he catch hell for that.

"Hey college boy." His words can only mean one thing.

Bill snaps around like a whiplash.

"You think you're so smart. Why can't you do what I tell you to do?

"I don't understand, sir."

"You fuck, you don't understand. How come you don't understand if you're so smart?"

"I don't know, sir."

"Now you've hit it ensign. Now we are in agreement. You don't know anything do you?"

Bill is silent.

"Do you," he screams.

Bill cannot answer. He slaps him hard. It stings and he is humbled.

"I'm not gonna take this shit from you ensign. You think you're smart, but what you don't seem to realize is that I know for a fact that you are stupid. I'm the one who's smart."

"Yes, sir."

"Now write these letters for me. Do you think you can handle that college boy?"

Bill takes the stack of papers.

"Yes, sir."

Good. He goes below where he belongs.

Out of nowhere the bomber comes, and the bullets fly through his legs. He is nailed to a wall of wind. His head turns forever. He has to let go of the papers. Out of the corner of his eye he sees them fly into the mask of God. They swirl like moths into a jet stream then dive into the sea. He cannot move his head.

If you want to think beach boss, think Robert Duvall in *Apocalypse Now* on the beach with his shirt off and his cowboy hat on—bullets firing all around him—he's impervious, barking locations to artillery on the destroyers. If you want to think my father as beach boss, think Robert Duvall as Boo Radley on the beach, or folded behind a door in Jem's room in *To Kill a Mockingbird*. Boo stands in a corner "leaning against the wall," hands sickly white "leaving greasy sweat streaks on the wall," pants stained, cheeks "thin to hollowness," eyes colorless gray, hair "dead and thin"—BUT he still saves the lives of Scout, the narrator, and her brother, Jem. Boo, shy and innocent, who doesn't live in the world, sticks a kitchen knife up under the ribs of Tom Ewell, the kind of man "you have to shoot before you can say hidy to 'em." Boo makes soap dolls for Scout and Jem, and what Scout gives in return is the narrative of their lives together, with Boo as the invisible hero. At the end of the novel, Scout becomes Boo, standing in his shoes and walking around in them, seeing the neighborhood and her own history from his angle. The vision makes her feel old.

What do Joseph Cornell, Theodore Kaczynski (the Unabomber), and my father have in common? This is a trick question. My father was not a terrorist but he was, like Kaczynski, a gifted man who became damaged by war. Ted became damaged at the hands of a psychiatrist at Harvard engaged in experiments on behalf of the military, experiments to see how much cruelty a sensitive human being could absorb without crumbling to pieces. Bill and Ted both flunked the experiment: they couldn't absorb the cruelty without consequence. Joseph Cornell became an artist who, having returned from Phillips

Academy, never left his home in Flushing, New York, the home he shared with his mother and younger brother Robert, also an artist, who suffered from cerebral palsy.

My father, Ted, and Joe are all descendants of Boo—not from Boo as he is in the novel, though, I suppose, partly, but descended from Boo as executed by Duvall in the film of Harper Lee's novel. Recovering from a laparascopic colon resection in 2005, I wrote an article for a Norwegian magazine issue dedicated to Don DeLillo. I noticed a certain Boo-like pattern in some of DeLillo's characters: ashen, fading, tender, pale, childlike. Don told me he had never read the novel. It doesn't matter. At that time, I still couldn't see the connection to my father. I had already written about the connection between Kaczynski and Cornell in the book I wrote with my husband, *Crimes of Art + Terror*. Then, at the Smithsonian in New York, all the men crashed together into focus. Maybe it was the picture of Cornell sitting in the backyard of his home in Flushing. The museum was showing some of his diary entries, letters, photographs. Something about his face as he sat in the chair looking out at whomever was taking the picture. The way my father used to look out the big picture window into the backyard of our house on Suffolk Avenue in Westchester, Illinois, traveling in his mind. Cornell's jagged handwriting looks like my father's postsurgical Parkinsonian scrawl. Despite the tremor he always wrote with his right hand.

After my father died we packed the garage with his extensive collection of 78 records: from Stravinsky's *Firebird Suite* to Rachmaninoff to his favorite, Oscar Peterson, the Maharaja of the keyboard. He loved to listen to music, the better to be alone with his thoughts. See the garage as a life-size Cornellian box.

Cornell kept dossiers on actresses, dancers, and singers with whom he had relationships—imaginary, real, or both. Had my father kept dossiers, had he been an artist as he had wanted, or as I like to imagine he wanted, he would have kept dossiers on Laurette Taylor, Benny Goodman, Oscar Peterson, Stravinsky, Horowitz. I remember he told me he heard Horowitz play, but that was probably before Bill got married. Horowitz blew Bill's mind.

Cornell loved ballet, music, and theater; so did my father. But he never went to the theater or to hear music, even though he worked in

Chicago. He dreamed of Tahiti but never went there. Maybe he's in Tahiti now, traveling in his mind.

Apocalypse

Whenever I ask Bill about Notre Dame he smiles wryly and says he was one of the Four Horsemen. Of course I believe him; I didn't know who they were except that my father was one of them. He makes no mention of their role, and thereby his role, in the apocalypse, though the apocalypse juxtaposes revelation and concealment, a favorite penchant of my father's, not unlike his claim of who he had been at Notre Dame. He was only writing, doing what he always liked to do. Meanwhile, a sports writer named Grantland Rice had already catapulted four sophomores into that myth: "Outlined against a blue, gray October sky the Four Horsemen rode again. In dramatic lore they are known as famine, pestilence, destruction and death. These are only aliases. Their real names are: Stuhldreher, Miller, Crowley and Layden [and McAuliffe, the invisible fifth wheel]. They formed the crest of the South Bend cyclone before which another fighting Army team was swept over the precipice at the Polo Grounds this afternoon as 55,000 spectators peered down upon the bewildering panorama spread out upon the green plain below." The year was 1924—my father was four years old. When the boys, all under six feet and none more than 162 pounds, returned from New York to South Bend and the glittering golden dome, they posed on horseback for a photo that fixed their fame forever in the annals of sports history. Bill could have told me he was anybody, but he chose to be one of them. No wonder he lamented that he couldn't throw the ball around with us. Must have been because of the surgery, though he never said and we never asked. I did hear one story about Notre Dame from my mother: my father had an issue with alcohol when he first went away to college, so much so that my grandmother talked to the priest at St. Edmund's to get Bill to stop drinking. He'll stop shortly after he marries, because of the medication, the phenobarbital.

For six months of training, he attends Midshipmen's School at Notre Dame, and Communications and Amphibious Tag in Virginia, where his sister Mary visits him. She notices him blinking a lot. He complains of feeling as if there were sand in his eyes—a neurological symptom. She insists that he should have been rejected for service, but he ships out to San Diego and the South Pacific.

I was an admiral in the Japanese navy, my father tells us, and we're starting to get the joke. We tell the Peterson boys next door that Dick McAuliffe, who played shortstop and second base at the time for the Detroit Tigers, was our father. We also tell the Marcy boys across the street that our mother could beat up their father, because our father, postsurgery, couldn't have beaten up anybody, despite his undisclosed high school boxing career. Fantasyland gets so bad at one point that my cousin Susie, after my father convinced us all to go with him on a safari to Basutoland (now known as Lesotho)—we didn't take much convincing, it was all a done deal—Susie goes home and cries to her father, Uncle Bob, begging to go with us. Even today, my brother didn't know Basutoland was a real country; he thought it was made up like everything else. Of course we never did go: the anticipation was all. Bill made the safari sound so wonderful, so much so that when I apply to college I want to study abroad in Africa, a dream doomed to die hard. Although, or because, my father could no longer hold his head straight, somehow he had not lost his sense of humor.

Tarawa

Brother Jack: *I think he* [Dad] *had battle fatigue from the war. I mean we know that because he had torticollis and we know where he was and we know what was going on there. It was not an uncommon thing. He was in the Gilbert Islands in 1943 and he had a bad relationship with his captain. I have to stop.*

Jack, overwhelmed, tears up and pulls away. Everything goes to hell inside of him right off the bat. The war defines him, too, in some unforgivable way, and he was never in it. Once he told me that he wished he'd been in a war: he wished he'd had that kind of life-defining challenge. Having it by proxy is not the same. Hell, maybe it's even worse. For Uncle Jack, my brother's spiritual father, the one he identifies with, the war was opportunity, escape, and the path to success.

It made him tough, tough enough to live ten years beyond what the doctors predicted when he was diagnosed with invading, destroying, squamous cell cancer. Tough enough to keep golfing even after disfiguring surgeries, his face half gone. Each time I see him, a little more of his head has been eaten away by the cancer until, finally, he looks as if a big chunk of his head has been blown clean off, but he's alive. He never turns his face away. He makes death fight for every inch of his body like an invading force on a South Pacific beach. You know that if he'd been at Tarawa he'd have survived intact. If my dad is Robert Duvall as Boo Radley, then Uncle Jack is Duvall as Lieutenant Colonel Kilgore on the beach in *Apocalypse Now*—hell, surfing the Nung River. It took the sun to finally beat Uncle Jack down, a tropical sun that brooked no mercy on the fair-haired boys from Oak Park.

Brother Jack (continuing): *There was a fundamental weakness that was with him* [Dad] *as a child. He was weak, he was sickly and subject to illness, and the family rallied to protect him. He was both physically and psychologically, to some extent, weak. Having said that I don't think there is a psychological makeup to withstand combat circumstances to which they were subject. On an LST, which is Landing Ship Tank, more commonly referred to as Large Slow Target, Dad was the communications officer, he was an ensign, he was the junior officer on board the ship. The captain was an old merchant marine, sea salt, didn't like him. Uneducated, coarse, tough, he believed in stern discipline for the men. The enlisted men stayed separate from the officers, and if an officer came to get rations or anything he went to the front of the line. Dad was well liked among the crew and didn't necessarily agree with that class system. He was very polite and the guy didn't like that. Furthermore, I think he was not exhibiting leadership qualities that were desired by the military at the time, or at any other time, which includes forcing the men to do things and so forth. So in all fairness, he was not necessarily suited for promotion.*

In any case, the tradition aboard the LST is to send the junior officer to the beach in a Higgins boat, that everyone sees in the movies where the front falls down, as a beach master. The beach master cannot hide with the marines, the beach master has to stand with the radio and observe everything that's going on on the beach, direct traffic and direct artillery—gunfire from the naval ships to the beach, in order to support the infantry. In the same way that artillery would support infantry in a land battle, the navy guns provide artillery support in an amphibious invasion. After Guadalcanal, which was the first amphibious assault, they were able to pretty much establish a beachhead. Certainly there was brutal fighting, but not during the initial landing. They were able to get established on the beach, move inland, and then proceed to take over the island.

Prior to Tarawa there had never been an amphibious assault that was contested. They wanted the Gilbert Islands because they wanted to encircle Rabaul, which was a large Japanese base. So they needed to establish bases around it and they didn't know—they knew that there was coral in the area of the landing—but they didn't know how deep it was, and a Higgins boat needs four feet of draft. As it happens, the coral was three feet deep. They couldn't land the Higgins boats and they had to stop some seven hundred yards from the beach. They did use what they call alligators. They did an intense shelling of Tarawa prior to the invasion and they grossly underestimated the Japanese ability to conceal and fortify their defenses. When they bombed, the sand from the explosions would land on top of the fortifications and strengthen them. So it was actually having a negative effect on the invasion. They [the Japanese] *zeroed the beach landing area because they knew about the coral and they knew what was going to happen when the marines would land. They basically massacred the marines when they landed. The beach master would have had to go on shore with the marines and then come back with the remains and/or wounded, but during the landing had to stay in charge of everything and stay alert and all that. It was the most dangerous job on the beach and certainly probably about the least pleasant. They gave it to the junior officer because in war the general consensus is that people that are the newest are the most expendable, because they have the least experience. A lot of people were mowed down. This was the genesis of the Navy SEALs who were to do underwater mapping. They would have gone to Tarawa surreptitiously, mapped the depth of the coral in order to prevent that in the future.*

There was a discrepancy in the obituary that said that he was in the invasion of the Marshall Islands, Guam, and Tinian and Saipan. The invasion of the Marshall Islands was subsequent to Tarawa—it was in 1944—and I had seen some medical records when Mom died that didn't jibe with the history. I remember Bob McAuliffe saying that Bill was in the Gilbert Islands. He's the one that told me he was a beach master. I had never been told that before and Bob said that was the worst job in the war (1991 or thereabouts when I went over to Bob's house—but he wasn't talking to me on that day, so let's say 1988 or so). Being sort of a war historian I compared the dates and saw that it didn't jibe. I think Mary just sort of had fantasies that he was in a more famous invasion. Tarawa is less known, but certainly very costly. As they went through the islands, as they got closer to Japan, more people died, Iwo Jima being the most notorious. Okinawa was the last one and by far the worst.

Tarawa was in November of 1943 and he was sent home in January of 1944. He could have been in a hospital in Honolulu. There was some talk of an incident where a fifty-caliber gun was shot between his legs. He mentioned that once. He thought that was the problem. Five inches, that's the diameter. It's not even a bullet, it's more like a shell; it's a small cannon. Friendly fire. It was onboard the ship. It was an accidental discharge or they happened to be shooting at something and he was in the wrong place at the wrong time. That's when he got torticollis.

Torticolly

It was Rabelais, a doctor, who first used the term tortycolly in a novel. Somebody gets his head cut off in a battle and somebody else, who hates tortycollys—hypocrites—worse than death, sews it back on for him, fitting vein to vein, muscle to muscle, nerve to nerve, and bone to bone. Neck surgery works better as satire. Rabelais's translator Burton Raffel translates tortycolly as "one of those hunched-over people." However, a hunchback is a very different thing than a tortycolly. Henri Bergson, in his analysis of comedy, argues that a hunchback is a man "bent on cultivating a certain rigid attitude whose body, if one may use the expression, is one vast grin." Certain deformities do not possess what Bergson calls the sorry privilege of causing some persons to laugh. He arrives at the following law: A deformity that may become comic is a deformity that a normally built person could successfully imitate.

Bergson sees a hunchback as someone who holds himself badly, contracted into an ugly stoop, someone who is physically obstinate, rigid, persistent, habitually contracted. One vast grin. In one of the most memorably terrifying horror films of my youth, another bad B-movie that [mis]shaped my consciousness—*Mr. Sardonicus*—a greedy grave robber's face is frozen into a hideous grin. The image of this grin imprints itself on my childish brain. The name Sardonicus alludes to a Sardinian plant which when eaten was supposed to produce convulsive laughter ending in death. In the movie, badly adapted from a 1961 modern gothic short story, it's not a plant, but the sight of his dead father's head that freezes the son's beautiful face into a death mask. More than the sight of his father's face, it's the knowledge that he's violating his father's grave to recover a winning lottery ticket that locks his jaw. Perhaps it's the idea that the shock of seeing something and the guilt of committing an immoral act can lock the body into some unnatural position that captures my imagination: what my father saw and/or did in the war turned his face forever. The image of Sardonicus is the image of death in life. The dead father lives—reanimated, replicated in the son. Or daughter.

This is the subconscious terror I grow up with—I will end as my father.

All the money in the world can't save the son from the hysterical consequences of his perfidious act of desecration. Sardonicus forces his beautiful wife's ex-boyfriend to perform a dangerous experimental procedure to cure him, or he will torture his wife—he's been doing this for years anyway. Injecting his face with a diluted poisonous plant extract that relaxes muscles in order to unfreeze his face, the doctor succeeds. The only thing is it's not really an experimental substance. It's only water, designed to cure his mind and thereby his body. The doctor and the beautiful wife run away together, and Mr. Sardonicus, still subconsciously determined to punish himself, discovers he can't open his mouth and starves to death. The deserted, emaciated Sardonicus, his mind shattered, roams his village searching for what my father liked to call "outside help." I see this picture on television probably when I am nine, the year when everything starts happening to me. My father's torticollis, my Uncle Jack's postsurgical mask, and the face of Mr. Sardonicus: all three masks hover before me now, fading in and out of each other in my own personal B-movie. Suddenly I see the connection. It all makes sense, but I don't know what it means exactly—as in those strange dreams where all the pieces fall into place, but by the time I wake up I can't, for the life of me, remember how.

In the year immediately following my father's expiration, I play a hunchback, the Fraulein Doktor in Durrenmatt's *The Physicists*, as a senior in college. Given the choice between a psychotic hunchback who wants to rule the world and the lead in Lanford Wilson's *Hot L Baltimore*, naturally I choose the hunchback, the final nail in the coffin of my impulse to perform in front of people. Big surprise, the Fraulein Doktor is the head of a mental hospital that houses three brilliant physicists as patients: Einstein, Mobius—inventor of the strip that bears his name—and Newton. So even after an old left-shoulder football injury and before I freeze both my shoulders at age forty-five expending inordinate violence on tennis balls too often, too fast, too hard, I feel compelled to contort my upper torso into a shadow version of my father's torticollis.

Frozen shoulder is an overuse injury. W. R. Gowers—neurologist, pediatrician, researcher, and artist—says excessive use of the muscles is probably an occasional cause of torticollis. Uh-oh. After sports-medicine physical therapy, deep-tissue massage, and a full round—that's ten, count 'em—of Rolfing, I finally figure out that I need to change my way of moving or I will continue to reinjure myself. My Advanced Rolfer tells me I should try Feldenkrais; I need neural reprogramming. Moshe Feldenkrais—Russian physicist, judo expert, mechanical engineer—created this method that focuses on awareness of habitual neuromuscular patterns and rigidities, and discovery of new ways of moving. Me, Slavophile and blue belt in karate, and Feldenkrais—it's love at first sight. As a sophomore in college I joined the karate club. My Japanese sensei—a WWII veteran whose personal mythology included a battle in which he singlehandedly held off, or was it decimated, fifty opponents—greets me with a bow.

His eyes glittering like fire, he locks into me: Miss McAuliffe, you killer. He, he, he (he laughs).

I protest feebly: No, Sensei, I'm not a violent person.

He, he, he. You toughest girl in Evanston.

No, really.

He, he, he.

He sees me.

Thirty years later, I find my therapist by chance and persistence. She's in the process of moving, so she doesn't return my first call. On a whim, or an angel's secret prodding, I phone this elusive Feldenkrais lady again and this time I find her. The elfin powerhouse named Candy tells me that my tennis injuries are both gift and revelation: the frozen shoulder issue I have had with both shoulders is intimately related to torticollis. This scares the shit out of me. She wants to know the history of my body.

When I was sixteen years old, I separated my left shoulder playing flag football. In an all-girls Catholic school this game bears infinitely more than a passing resemblance to rugby, tackles and all. First leap into the black zone where I am merely a vessel with no will, only surrender; then catch the bomb from Janet T's golden fingers for a touchdown—a catch so impossible that the boys from the high school where I am a cheerleader tell me that they wish they had my hands; score. Still high on that floating slowed-down time, feeling invincible and wanting to test that theory, I click the decision to charge right into those four girls coming at me, plow right into them: I hear the crunch inside my body and, standing on the sidelines, I go into shock and spend six weeks in a sling.

Let's talk about that click: first time I must have felt it I am two and a half standing on the curb with a big car lumbering down Suffolk Avenue in slow motion in my mind. I am across the street from our house when my mother sees me click that decision—I decide I can run across the street and beat the car. She thinks she can't stop me and she's probably right—what else is new?— but I have to ask what am I doing alone on the opposite side of the street? How exactly did I get there at two and a half? The newspaper reports that I darted across the street and the "boat," belonging to Mrs. June M of the next street over, hits me. Reports indicate that the right front end of the car—I almost made it!—strikes me, and three stitches sewn by Dr. Forbrich, my pediatrician dubbed by me and my brothers Four-BrickHead, close the cut on the right side of my head. Desire to pun must be genetic.

Candy watches me move and tells me I am locked and loaded. After we've been working together for three years, Candy turns my head to the right: If only you could hold your head like that, everything would be fine. This puts the fear of God in me because my father's torticollis turned his head to the right. It makes me nervous even to hold my head like that, afraid maybe it will freeze like an ugly grimace. She calls this the elusive obvious and cites this as a major breakthrough in our work together. My father's body is in my body. This is how I keep him alive, how I keep him close.

Friday April 26, 1974 [third entry]

Today we had our little picnic on the terrace with our "shared living" group. We had fried chicken, potato salad, ice cream, coleslaw, +, all in all, very enjoyable to the last morsel. And to top everything else off Dr. Rovner came shortly before our last group therapy meeting after supper + said I could be discharged permanently after last week's successful weekend and could return to work Monday 4-29-74.

This gave me just the challenge I needed to continue my psychological recovery, although, the doctor told me, the psychological wedge had been driven into the block of uselessness, despair + insanity that has been gradually destroying my wife, my kids, and my friends + relatives there still remain many solid strokes of the axe to completely shatter the irrationality of all those previous weekends + holidays. Now I know I have the power to quell these attacks; to knock them in the bud, before they even get started.

Because I can successfully imitate my father's torticollis, is it funny? No one ever laughed at my father's rigidity though they stared, but I can imitate it—even if I'm afraid to do it. The ritual imitations my brother and I conduct never involve my father's torticollis, only his dementia. Scary/funny has always been an electric combination for me, almost as good as funny/sad.

My acting coach suggests I use upholstery webbing to wrap—under the crotch and over one shoulder, not without discomfort—and twist my already locked and loaded ribcage and post-traumatic shoulder into a lopsided hunch, right shoulder higher than the left, head leaning unfailingly, naturally, to the right. I study a hunchback librarian at the university library for hours on end, to build the physicalization for Fraulein Doktor, when all along my perfect model lies just beneath my skin like shingles waiting to erupt. One night, in the middle of the performance, I go up—theatre speak for I forgot my lines—and freeze in free fall, minus the blind dark pleasure of catching the bomb, feeling only blind terror. Afterward, one of my mentors cites that moment as my best: he could see me stop thinking. It is only now that I see this episode as a manifestation of my father's rigid fear in my nervous system. The frozen ghost hovers invisibly—waiting for the right moment to pop out, like a head with crazy hair popping down out of the attic. Years before, I saw *The Haunting* at my cousin's farm in Door County, Wisconsin, where my bed sat directly off the landing, complete with a trap door to the attic: the perfect setting to imagine the head of the crazy member of the family, relegated to the uninhabited upstairs, come tumbling down to scare me in the middle of the night.

On pre-confusion Saturday afternoons, Bill takes the three of us kids to the movies, in lieu of the much venerated (by him) tossing a ball around, what Dad perpetually lamented that he could not do, even though we professed not to care. The films I remember best from childhood are the ones I went to with my father, grade-B horror films and adult thrillers in which naked and almost-naked female bodies make cameo appearances: *Goldfinger*, with the girl's naked body painted gold, *Dr. Strangelove*, and *The Spy Who Came in from the Cold.* The plot sufficiently beyond me— I'm not alone in this—I take fascinated notice of an obscure woman stripping in the background of a club. In *Haunted Palace*, the kids with the clay patches where their eyes should be wander around like zombies. The sight of them makes me flee the dark cavern of the theater only to wander alone around the lobby of the Lido in Maywood, down the street from the A&W stand—root beer in a frosty mug for five cents. And let's not forget *Spartacus*: he gets crucified for leading a slave revolt, but his child is born free. *Spartacus* makes my little brother cry. Jack says Dad took us to films we shouldn't have seen; he says his chronic lack of judgment in this area directly indicates his pathology. I think I thought it was cool. I guess I still do, even though I was so scared of the giant squid in *Twenty Thousand Leagues under the Sea* that I wanted to flee the theater. I couldn't move. Did I know even then, at ten years old, that there was a monster lurking in the blind depths of my very own house? Under the bed, in the toilet, in the closet, on the door, or in the room next door where my parents sleep. I must have thought it normal to be scared. Somebody get me some clay so I can cover my eyes.

I have the same bottomless experience of terror years later while drift diving off the coast of Cozumel, carried along by the current with my younger, and infinitely more experienced, brother. Both of my brothers became highly qualified divers, water their natural element. When I signal to him that I need to go up because I literally can't stay down, he gives me that look and shrugs with frustration, but relents and takes me up slowly, safely, to the surface. Then he finds somebody else to buddy with, someone willing and able to drift.

I do my drift diving in the theater.

July 3, 1973

Dear Jody,
I had intended writing you last Saturday, but, as usual, the day was a complete wipeout for me. Rescue finally came Sunday morning, though, in the sublime

ecstasy of reading the Sunday Tribune + hauling my degenerated carcass to Mass at Divine Infant Sunday morning.

Enough of my inequities for now. Let's talk about you. I was sorry to hear that you're not altogether happy at your current place of employment [as a singing waitress at a Michigan resort]. *But try + buck up, + if it gets too unbearable just pack up + come on home. You won't have any trouble getting a job around here.*

I know how you feel, though, honey, in wanting to get out + be on your own where you can think + reflect on the vicissitudes of life as it relates to your personal ego.

Just remember that I am always with you on your side of the fence. You are one of my very favorite people.

Love,
Dad

In June of 1944, Bill, stricken with torticollis (a.k.a. wry-neck), is in a hospital in Honolulu, reflecting on the vicissitudes of his life. Despite his injury, if we can call it that, from February 1944 to December 1945 he is still on active service. The navy doesn't discharge him because they are hoping against hope, one of my father's favorite phrases whose meaning eludes me even now, he'll be able to come back. He will never come back to life. Not to active service and not to who he was before the war. By the summer of 1945 he is stateside. The Notice of Separation bears my father's signature, in a notably tremor-less right-handed script. In September of 1945, Japan surrenders.

Gowers: *The prognosis must be grave in every developed case.*

In my father's case, he puts his left hand up to stop whatever is coming at him, then his head jerks to the right. Is his war-induced—if it is!—spasmodic torticollis, not fatal but disfiguring, an index of his sensitivity and passivity? To his doctor, his behavior invited blame and implied weakness, but Bill was stubborn—an inexplicable quality in a man so allegedly (one of Bill's favorite words) weak of will. Though Bill never mentions torticollis in his diary, his neurologist's assessments—a moral and psychological judgment—suggest that Bill fit the profile of a spasmodic torticollis character type, a type of personality considered especially susceptible.

In the midst of both world wars, there were torticollitics. During WWI, L. P. Clark describes torticollitics as having shrunk from their adult tasks in life and taken refuge in the simple, crude reaction—torticollis. They had suffered "nerve strain" and found relief in what he describes as an unfortunate disorder. Once they realize they cannot get rid of it by force of will, they lament. The bottom-line egregious offense here is WEAKNESS, and the exercise of WILL after onset is hopeless. In those days psychoanalysis was a last resort. Perhaps Bill should have received psychoanalysis immediately, but his or his family's need to see his problem as physical, not mental, prevented his family from supporting that approach. Though the exact mechanism for torticollis remains unknown, we know today that the cause stems from abnormal electrical activity. The network for voluntary movement is disturbed. I like to think of it as a mental monsoon—deep in the brain.

I never thought of my father as weak but, rather, as extremely strong-willed. Long before WWI, French neurologist Henry Meige (1866–1940), lumped these WEAKNESSES of so-called primary instincts—judgment, will, perception—under "mental infantilism." Such mental infants were indecisive, vacillating, weak-willed, or erratically brilliant, emotionally unstable persons, or both. Deprived of opportunities to express such erratic brilliance, they might exhibit it in their bodies. Dr. Meige would have prescribed writing in order to treat my father's torticollis.

I learn my father's movement pattern from Sally S, who loved my father. I called her, after I got her number from my brother, thinking I'd uncover some romance hidden in my father's past. I nurture hope that he may have had a great and secret love affair before my mother, and that this lover reveals herself to me at my mother's funeral, thirty years after my father has expired. But Sally is nine years old when she meets my father. Bill is twenty-four, having just returned from duty in the South Pacific.

The navy tells Bill not to go home, not to be near his mother. So he goes instead to Michigan City, where his family has the summer cottage, but he stays with Sally and her mother, a corporate client of Bill's father. Sally calls what Bill has a nervous tic.

Sally: *I knew him when I was nine years old. My memories of him? A wonderful man, troubled. My mother adored him. They played round robin with Dr. B in Michigan City. Mother made Bill welcome. We'd take walks. Your father's mother and Bill taught me how to play solitaire. He was very patient. He used to go for walks. He was kind, very troubled. He had a nervous tic: he put his hand up and his head would jerk. It got worse under stress. When he woke up in the morning it wasn't bad. He didn't talk to me about the war, he talked to my mom. Something about an LST blew up. I loved him so much it didn't matter. I didn't care. I asked my mother why does he do that. She told me he's shell shocked. He wrote a lot and went out for walks with the dogs, a couple of dachshunds. We'd go for long walks with the dogs.*

The malady known as spasmodic wry-neck is analogous to tic douloureux. In 1928, Dr. Clark defines a tic as "a coordinated purposive act, provoked in the first instance by some external cause or by an idea" and then perpetuated as a repetitive involuntary movement: a derangement of neural function occurring in the absence of organic nervous disease. According to Clark, the greatest fault in the ticeur's disorder is not in the movement but in the amount of isolation and banishment, which the mental torticollis engenders within him. The torticollitic becomes a truly obsessive individual and the tic is raised to a broad and deep habit of obsessive thinking. The stigma changes the identity of the sufferer. What seems to have happened is that during Bill's infamous ten-year death march, his spells constituted a kind of total tic, a turning away from work and family and a retreat deeper and deeper into an internal escape or confinement. He could not remember the Saturday episodes, the weekend episodes, the benders when the neuro-drunk blacks out. Tic in adults is apt to be one of the most intractable of functional nervous disorders.

Tic, tac, tag—he's it.

December 9, 1972

Dear Jody,
. . . It will be so nice to have you + Brien home for the holidays in the bosom of your family.

I don't know why I continuously resort to that above homily, but I can only conclude that it's due to brain fatigue which is an occupational hazard with us vocational counsellors. Comes from overworked brain activity during the week, coping with drunks, prostitutes + other unhappy individuals.

This note will have to terminate briefly as Joy has just stentorially announced the call to lunch + it may well be the last meal for me before my untimely demise.

I've decided that what is really bothering me is a rare malady known as Oxcart's syndrome which consists solely of being subjected to too many working days + too few holidays.

All kidding aside, though, darling, I really miss your vitriolic presence around here + will be very pleased to have you home for the holidays.

Take care of yourself, love.

Love,
Dad

Cancer patients don't run into the street in their underwear looking for "outside help." The insiders—us—are failing Bill. If his disease is a failure of will, then it's not dementia—it's a character flaw. Those of us in full-time contact with his on-again off-again dementia find it more difficult to accept him than, say, his sister and younger brother who knew him pre-torticollis, before the war, the first turning point in his short unhappy life. The surgery transforms him from a person with a stigma to a person with a corrected stigma. Later he becomes a person who sometimes passes as undemented. His neurologist achieves a radical reinvention of Bill's past as a series of overprotections and irresponsibilities. Bill buys his new identity whole cloth, but puts some of it in quotes, his theatrical sensibility persevering against all odds to the bitter end. The fact that his literary wit continued to function, even as he was losing his mind, made us think he might be losing it on purpose.

The condition of torticollis is rare under thirty, Bill's contracted at twenty-four. Malarial poison can cause spasm in the neck. My mother claimed he had a mild form of malaria, what she called cat fever, in the South Pacific, but, by all accounts except Mary's, he was a robust individual in perfect health when it came on.

Bill never complained of pain. My brother to this day considers Bill a victim of shell shock/battle fatigue/post-traumatic stress disorder, and the surgery a literally wrongheaded (as it were) mistake. He's surprised to hear from me that there are cases of torticollis that are not hysterical. Hysterical spasm spreads from the neck to the trunk, which becomes affected by writhing movements. In my father's case, conditions of onset—war—raised suspicion that his case might be hysterical in nature. It came on acutely, which is rare.

Sydenham: *When the Mind is disturb'd by some grevious* [sic] *Accident, the animal Spirits run into disorderly motions; the Urine appears sometimes limpid, and in great quantity; the sick persons cast off all hope of recovery. . . . Whatsoever part of the body the Disease doth affect (and it affecteth many) immediately the symptoms that are proper to that Part appear.*

Bill saw an LST blow up and looked away. It is, of course, ludicrous on a certain level to think that looking away from an exploding ship can provoke a neurological disorder. Yet, the typical hysterical case woke up one morning in his bunk and his head suddenly twisted over toward his left shoulder. He experienced a sharp pain in the right side of his neck, but his muscle was not in spasm. After receiving reassurance and anesthetic spray, plus encouragement to hold his head normally, the typical case returned to normal. No amount of reassurance or psychotherapy in the form of anesthetic spray could restore my father to normal.

Reassurance was a major word in my world growing up, from the time I was around ten years old until the time my father expired when I was twenty. Seemingly modest but inexorably persistent in his demands, he repeatedly asked us for just a little reassurance. The problem was that no amount of reassurance would suffice, and if you gave a little, he demanded more.

An hysteric was likely to show improvement when told that X-rays of his cervical spine are normal, that is, when he received the proper reassurance. It was important to rule out true organic lesions, associated trauma, or preceding illness or exposure. Dad's autopsy would show lesions.

On what would have been my father's eighty-ninth birthday, Donald T fender-bends me on the boulevard, and Candy says it's my Dad—a wake-up call from the dead zone—trying to get ahold of me. I respond with a torticollian tension in my head and neck. That's where my focus is these days. Dad had to wait for Donald T to get distracted so he could bump me, reminding me to call Erica C in the coroner's office in Chicago and keep trying to extract a copy of his mythical autopsy report. Erica's in charge of old autopsies, off-site, in some remote location. It takes me awhile to find her in the first place, but when I do she gives me her cell number and tells me to call her; she says she always has it with her. I call a couple of times, but only during business hours. The first time she picks up she's with her child at the doctor's. This feels too personal, as if I'm crossing some kind of boundary into Chicagoan Kafkaland. Maybe I'm already there. The second time she doesn't answer. I leave a businesslike message, but from here on out I'm calling the office whether she answers or not.

I remember the first time I read *The Metamorphosis* in high school: my father is just like Gregor Samsa. That makes me the sister, who grows irritable taking care of the monster that once was her beloved brother. Unable to put up with the constant torture at home, she finally pounds her fist on the table and decides to get rid of it. Otherwise, her mother will die. It's my mother who tells me, at twenty years old, that I have to commit my father to an institution. That's right, me. The situation is killing her. The sister's own movements turn mechanical. Her neck stiffens like her brother's. She insists the insect is not her brother. If it were, he would have gone off to die. She locks him in his room for the last time, though it's hardly necessary for he cannot move at all now. Dusty fluff covering the rotten apple his father threw at him—long since embedded in his inflamed, but no longer painful, back—he thinks back on his family with deep emotion and love. They lock Bill in Ward 51B and forget all about him. He knows eminently well (my father's words) that he has to disappear. When the time comes, his head, like Gregor's, must sink to the floor in death WITHOUT HIS CONSENT. Kafka was right about everything. At the end, the sister gets up and stretches her young body, full of life, her future wide open. Time to find a good husband. Or maybe she will wake up one morning from unsettling dreams . . .

After waiting three months for the autopsy report from Cook County, I get a form in the mail from Erica C. After an extensive search, the record of death could not be located. The death of my father was classified a NAMEC—Not A Medical Examiner's Case. I will need to contact the hospital where the autopsy was performed. I talk to a live person, Tracy E, at Hines who calls me back the same day with information. She has, she says, good news and bad news. The bad news is that the only vestige of his existence at Hines is what's called a 3x5 Locator Card. The good news is that the Locator Card bears a stamp that indicates that Bill's records had been shipped to the VA Regional Office. This means that I can write to the Privacy Officer to see what I can recover. I have only to send a copy of the death certificate and a copy of my driver's license. On the Locator Card are the dates of his two stays at Hines: 1) November 27, 1954–December 31, 1954, and 2) June 16, 1975–August 26, 1975. On both occasions he was in Ward 51B. I can tell that Tracy doesn't know how I will handle the information that he was in Ward 51B. She's been around long enough to remember that 51B is a psychiatric ward, one of four in a cluster of what were, at that time, psych buildings. She gently explains that it could have been for substance abuse as well as mental illness, as if drug rehab is better than mental rehab. She doesn't know how much I know about my father's case, that I actually visited him in the ward. When I ask her if she knows the circumstances under which a patient would be sent to Downey, she chuckles because she's one of the few around anymore who remembers that North Chicago Medical Center was once called Downey, as in going down for the count. She's been there for thirty years. A patient would have been sent there because Downey was then and is now a domiciliary, set up to take care of veterans for longer terms—three months to a year. When I call back a few minutes later to confirm the dates, she insists that he was only at Hines once, but consents to get the card and check. She admits that I was correct and I see just how elusive my history really is. I need to confirm the dates because the dates are my own private Rorschach. November 27 means that my father said he wanted to jump out the Mercy Hospital window on November 26, two days after I was born. My mother gave birth to me the day before my father had experimental neurosurgery. What in the hell (my mother's expression) were my parents thinking! My mother and I went home from the hospital and my father did not return home until December 31, 1954. And all that time, through Christmas Day, he was in the psychiatric ward, with my mother and two babies at home. When I ask to get a copy of the Locator Card, Tracy tries to dissuade me, explaining that I will have to send copies of my father's death certificate, my driver's license, my birth certificate, and my mother's death certificate, because she was my father's next of kin at the time of his death. It seems more complicated to get that card than get the records, or what's left of them, from the VA Regional Office.

I'm still waiting for the autopsy report. When I tell my brother I'm trying to recover it, he says good luck. I could die waiting. Kafka rules.

> For an analogy in the literature of antiquity to the modern sense of a shaming, isolating disease, one would have to turn to Philoctetes and his stinking wound.
>
> — SUSAN SONTAG, *Illness as Metaphor*

My father goes to graduate school in playwriting at the University of Hawaii on the GI Bill, and I go to graduate school in directing at the Yale School of Drama. My teacher tells us we all have only one idea, one story to tell, and the trick is finding different ways to tell it. When I reflect on the question of whether or not there is a singular idea that has driven my post-hunchback theater work as a director, I must acknowledge the theme of the deteriorating male figure in almost all the plays I chose to direct: Don DeLillo's *Mao II*—Bill Grey, reclusive failed writer, in quest of the lost creativity he felt as a child, gets hit by a car and dies anonymously on a freighter steaming to Beirut; Neal Bell's *McTeague*—his vocation lost, the lottery won, greed born, he ends up dead in the desert handcuffed to his erstwhile friend; Tennessee Williams's *Orpheus Descending*—a man with a guitar tries to save his Eurydice, ends up burned alive; Strindberg's *The Father*—the inventor, unhinged by doubts about his fatherhood, ends up in a straitjacket; Leonid Andreyev's *He Who Gets Slapped*—an intellectual hides in the circus, becomes a clown, commits murder, and ends up a suicide.

Deteriorating males, usually artist figures, compel me.

Bertolt Brecht's *Drums in the Night*—my thesis production at Yale—

is the story of a dead soldier who comes back from the grave to get his girl back. I cast a man named Bill—Catholic, guilt-ridden, tending toward depression, brilliant artist, true friend and kindred spirit who will die young in real life—as Kragler, the German soldier who returns from war in Africa having dug his way out of his own grave. Kragler, the ever-bleeding hero, drafted into the Spartacist revolt in postwar Germany, refuses his role, grabs his girl—pregnant by a war profiteer who stayed home—and embraces his big, broad, white bed. He takes off his uniform and multiplies, so he will not perish from the earth. That's the way to go.

My mother turns to me after the performance, my father dead five years at this point. He looks just like Bill, she says: this, after I had Kragler cut his own hair so that he'd look as if he'd been a POW. This comes as news to me, because my capacity to consciously put two and two together when it comes to my father is clearly compromised. The elusive obvious strikes again. Why Kragler? I guess I needed to see my father again, find out, at long last, what happened in the war. I wanted him to get the girl. I wanted him to claw his way out of his grave and come back to me, or I'd have to keep reinventing him on the stage.

The Haunting

The theme of the revenant, the one who returns from death—like Kragler in *Drums in the Night*—has haunted me since I was a child.

It's 1964 and I'm nine years old; my cousin Cindy, whom I love, is eight—she's in the grade behind me. Her older sister is Debbie. Soon my father will tell me that he'll die in ten years.

My family is sitting in the kitchen. It's Saturday, the day when things will start falling apart in my house. The phone rings and I answer it. It's my Uncle Bob, my father's younger brother. He says, Hello, is your mother there? I think he sounds funny.

I know they're on vacation out West, visiting dude ranches and national parks. My mother gets on the phone. He says, Debbie and Cindy are dead. They were murdered. He says, Joy, I'm calling you because I know you're strong and you'll be able to bear the burden for the rest of the family.

My mother thinks he's crazy. We can't believe it. My father starts crying, the first time I ever see him cry. I don't know what it means that they're dead. I think—Oh, they'll come back. I'll have three wishes and one of them will be that Debbie and Cindy will come back.

I remember my aunt and uncle were in a hotel in Jackson Hole, Wyoming, at a floor show with the Smothers Brothers, but when I search the *Chicago Tribune* archives I discover they were in a motel lobby watching television. Twelve-year-old Debbie, Cindy, and six-year-old Susie were all in the same room upstairs; I think Debbie and Cindy in the double bed. Cindy has a fever that night and Aunt Betty almost stays with her.

An itinerant dishwasher named Pixley (a.k.a. Armandoz) climbs to the roof and removes the screen to break in. Busted for kiting checks two years earlier, this future murderer entered the army and the charge was dropped. Less than a month before this "smiley, quiet" loner commits double murder of two of Bob's three young daughters, he steals a car, gets stopped by police, but manages to talk his way out of it, convincing them that he was "only a passenger and not involved" in the theft.

I remembered that Uncle Bob heard screams so he went up the stairs and he caught this drifter named Pixley, but in reality they had heard nothing. The paper says that when they came to check on the girls, they found Pixley on the floor beside or between the dead girls, drunk or asleep, or feigning drunkenness or sleep. Bob holds him until Policeman Jensen arrives at the scene of the crime to arrest Pixley, whose only words are "I didn't do this. I didn't do this."

Bob said, "Susan sat up in her bed, blinking as tho she had been asleep." I had always imagined that she must have hidden, maybe under the bed, like Cora A who escaped Richard Speck, as the other eight nurses, held for hours and systematically raped and killed one by one, waited, paralyzed in dread of the inevitable. I read that Pixley bludgeoned Debbie with a heavy rock which was found in the room, strangled Cindy, and raped them after they were dead.

County Attorney Floyd King said: "Surprisingly Pixley's clothing was not bloody. An examination of his body, however, showed dried blood on his underclothing. There seems little doubt that he killed and then molested these children." I didn't know what that meant at the time. My brother says the law won out in Bob's mind when he didn't kill him with his bare hands. If he had killed him right then—instead of throttling him and holding him on the floor until the cops pulled him off—nobody would have blamed him. His life might have turned out differently, better. He might have felt differently about himself, felt something other than that he should have saved them. He couldn't help but feel that he should have saved them. He might have felt that at least he avenged them.

My aunt went to the county jail to look at Pixley. She talked to him through the window of his cell: "I'm the mother of those girls; I'm their mother." He was leaning against the wall some eight feet away with a blank stare on his face. She said: "I hope you get the electric chair for what you did to my babies. I'll never forget what they looked like when you finished with them."

My youngest cousin survived. On the stand in open court pleading innocent by reason of insanity, the defendant, who claimed he'd been in an alcoholic blackout, said that if he had known she was there he would have killed her, too. So Uncle Bob did save Susie, his youngest child. Pixley got the gas chamber.

They said they felt a sense of kinship with all the parents who have lost their children—the Grimes sisters, two girls who disappeared in Chicago and were later found dead in a ditch with a thin layer of ice covering their naked bodies, the younger one molested; Judith Mae Anderson, her remains found in an oil drum in Lake Michigan; the Peterson-Schuessler boys, found naked and dead, and all the rest. "We have been spared the ordeal of other parents—of going through life, looking into the eyes of strangers, and wondering 'Could this be the one who did it?'" As far as I could tell, they had been spared nothing.

I'm not permitted to go to the wake or the funeral: my mother thinks my presence will upset my aunt. So close to them in age, I'll remind her of them. In a recurring dream they appear at our back door and say, We're back. I can see them through the screen. They want to come in, but they never do. So close in life, they're buried in death in the same casket in the cold mausoleum, because my aunt cannot bear to put their bodies into the ground. This is so they won't be alone in Paradise, wearing matching add-a-pearl necklaces—my grandmother gave me one, too. It's lost before I ever have a chance to add any pearls. My mother sends me to the home of her best friend from nursing school, Loretta. I watch *The Headless Horseman* on television.

Terrified not only of the headless man, but also of what I don't know, I go to bed alone with a huge hopeless crush on Loretta's older-than-me son.

The yellowed, brittle newspaper clippings recording the event, subsequent trial, and execution of the killer, the last to die in the gas chamber in Wyoming, lie buried in the buffet under a green glass bowl that only comes out for company. Of course I find them and read them, even though or because I'm not supposed to, the secret story I'm not supposed to know. The clippings, long since disintegrated, are buried in the vault of my head for good. Many years later my mother assails me with a concrete detail: when my uncle discovers the killer in the room with his two dead children, the killer is still on top of the younger one, the one I loved, with his naked ass showing. My uncle has to pull him off of her and somehow manages not to kill him. The papers didn't tell the whole story. I don't need to know that fact, and now I see it like I was there. The killer smashes her face in with a rock. To stop her screaming, my mother says.

I couldn't take in the fact that they were dead until about five years after it happened. My surviving cousin and I got to be pretty close. I always thought I'd ask her how she survived, but I could never do it until after my mother died. At my mother's wake—my mother's death in the room gave me license—she said that her parents got her therapy right away and it helped her. Children are more resilient than adults.

Bob and Betty lived in Maywood, a predominantly black middle-class neighborhood with neat rows of houses, the hometown of many of the soldiers who endured or failed to endure the notorious Bataan Death March. Bob's death march starts in Jackson Hole and leads to a grave in Chicago. I assume my uncle lost whatever faith he'd had in God. Sometimes I noticed my Uncle Bob looking at me with particular intensity. Then he'd ask me how old I was. I knew what he was thinking then, what they would look like if they had lived. Would they look like me? So my mother was right. Seeing me was painful.

For years the murders haunt Bob—great judge but bad businessman, says Uncle Jack—and eventually contribute to the severe depression from which he suffered. Prompted by personal and financial hardship brought on by bad investments, he resigns voluntarily from the bench in 1979, after he's found unfit. By then he has a new family in addition to his first wife and surviving daughter. After losing Debbie and Cindy, he meets somebody new and they conceive a son whom I have never met. Bob enters into a professional relationship with an attorney who specializes in personal injury work. Within less than a year his partner is disbarred, so he enters into a similar relationship with his former partner's attorney.

Around that time, for reasons not part of the public record, his son moves with his mother to California and Bob visits them regularly. The attorney terminates their partnership and refuses to pay him. Distraught over his financial situation and suffering from what a psychologist called neurotic depression, Bob files complaints against the attorney. Court documents concerning these complaints tell me that Bob's mental condition deteriorates and he becomes obsessed by the fear that his son would be violently murdered as two of his daughters had been seventeen years before. Having stopped bathing and dressing properly, he goes to his son's school every day just to make sure he's still alive. When his son's mother asks him to leave, he returns to Chicago.

Back in Chicago, he suffers two heart attacks, the second one massive. Having lost seventy-five pounds, he thinks he's going to die. Suffering from major psychotic depression, he admits himself to a state psychiatric institute for treatment, but can't be treated because of his heart condition. He leaves the hospital against medical advice and suffers a third heart attack that very day.

Convinced that his death is imminent, he agrees to a settlement with his former partner in exchange for recanting the charges and statements he had made against him. Intent on returning to his son so he can see him one last time before he dies, he signs what his counsel warns are "horrible" documents (because recanting sworn testimony), without reading them. As soon as he gets the money, he sets out for California, driving alone. Somewhere in Wyoming—I imagine somewhere near Jackson Hole—he loses consciousness and is hospitalized for a time. He's trying to get to his son, but his soul has its own agenda. He needs to lose consciousness near the place where he lost his first two children.

In 1982, he's admitted to a VA hospital for treatment of a coronary condition and psychiatric problems. During the hospitalization, he's assigned to the "Brain-Damaged Ward," where he receives antidepressant drugs. After this treatment, his physical and emotional health greatly improves. He returns to work. Somewhere in here my mother loans him money, more than once. She knows she'll never get it back, but she wants to help him. After all, Bob was there for my father when he needed help, and life has brought Bob to his knees. The court holds that censure is the appropriate sanction for recanting a sworn statement. The judgment is merciful, taking into account what the court considered extraordinary mitigating circumstances. "Extraordinary mitigating circumstances" hardly begins to describe what happened. Had he killed Pixley on the spot, he would have had a "normal" life—sort of.

I'm connecting the dots now, between the murders and my father's revelation to me that he will die in ten years, between the beach at Tarawa and a motel room in Jackson Hole, between the Brain-Damaged Ward and Building 51, both at the VA. The tragic record of Bob's life—different from but as damning as my father's—starts to work its way into the fiber of the play of my father's life. The debased Pixley, for whom there is and can be no compassion, has entered the nauseating, dramatically moving spectacle. This is when I start thinking people want to kill me. As I told you before, I do have my reasons. Later my shrink will tell me that in most cases this irrational fear is a function of general anxiety, but in my case, this thought is rational. My mother and grandmother, determined that I should not meet the same fate, teach me to be afraid. My parents get me a dog. On the street, I avoid eye contact if I think somebody coming toward me is iffy, cross the street when necessary, and pretend to be mental on the "L" as required.

Miss McAuliffe, you killer. You toughest girl in Evanston. He, he, he.

Years later, when I go to the mausoleum at Queen of Heaven cemetery, I cannot find their tomb.

The last time I talk to Uncle Bob is over the telephone, when I'm considering law schools in Chicago, and Bob advises me against the University of Chicago. He says, if you want to practice law, don't go to the University of Chicago. That was 1991 and he lived until 1998, a good seventeen years after 1981, when he thought he was doomed. I remember the day he dropped dead of a heart attack on a Chicago sidewalk. I thought, that's how I'd like to go—out like a light. But he didn't go out like a light. Far from it. Like my father, his life got smaller and smaller, slowly and painfully, long before the lights went out.

Why can't we be like the Waltons, my father laments. Goodnight, Johnboy.

Goodnight, Brien. Goodnight, Jody. Goodnight, Jack. Goodnight, Joy.

A Cloud of Vultures

Fast forward to the early 80s and I'm living in the West Village with two male roommates, one of whom professes to love me, though he's mostly not there. When he's not there he's mostly having sex with other women, of which I am not aware. Maybe there's a darkness behind my eyes at the time: being with me is like driving by a cemetery. I cry a lot late at night, and he doesn't want to comfort me. In search of a direct descendant of *Drums in the Night*—because I've only just begun to get the ghost out of my system—I am led, seemingly inexorably, to *Philoctetes* by Heiner Müller, a contemporary version of the story of the great archer with the stinking foot. Honey, it's the new Müller!—our running gag about my noncommercial play choice, Müller not exactly a household name in New York. Philoctetes ships out for Troy, but en route a water snake bites him, leaving him with a reeking wound that refuses to heal. The Greeks cannot win without him and his bow, and Odysseus must trick him into returning to the Trojan War.

Bill, in San Diego before shipping out to the South Pacific and Tarawa, bitten by a neurological snake, blinks repeatedly, as if there were sand in his eyes.

The intolerable stench from Philoctetes's festering wound makes him a pariah. The Greeks, who can't stand listening to his crying, stick him on the island of Lemnos, where he stays until they need him in order to win the war.

The Navy takes torticollitic Bill out of action. His wound doesn't smell, but it can spread like hysteria, like fear itself.

Odysseus, who left Philoctetes on Lemnos in the first place, returns with Neoptolemus, son of Achilles. Philoctetes, consumed by hatred, no longer himself, resists returning with those who abandoned him.

Bill, no longer himself, consumed by guilt not hatred, his torticollis no longer acute but chronic, never returns to the front. His older brother encourages him to return to Oahu five years after the war ends, but the vultures have begun to gather behind his eyes.

In East German Müller's version of the play, Neoptolemus has to kill Philoctetes to protect Odysseus, the leader, and the future of Greece. The ever practical Odysseus carts the corpse of Philoctetes back to Troy and victory: a dead Philoctetes is better than no Philoctetes at all. This is, after all, a Commie version of the tale.

The same Bill who played Kragler plays Philoctetes. You see the pattern. When my mother comes to see the production in New York, she tells me how proud my father would have been, if only he had lived to see me direct a play in New York.

A few years later, I trek uptown to the Thalia to see *Let There Be Light*, John Huston's documentary about battle fatigue in WWII. John Savage's twitchy—he's always twitchy—reenactment, in Andrei Konchalovsky's film *Maria's Lovers*, alerts me to the original. There's Bill, on the big screen in the all-but-deserted art house, in living black and white, not Bill himself, but others like him—what the voiceover calls "human salvage," shadows on the side of the destroyer as they walk the plank to a stint in a psychiatric facility on the long road home. Can they ever go home again? *Look Homeward, Angel*, one of my father's favorite books, says no. White tags clipped to their shirt pockets, cigarettes and fear of death unite them. None of Huston's subjects has torticollis, but they tremble, stutter, can't sleep, can't remember, suffer mental pains—including a case of conversion hysteria, purely psychological paralysis. Huston shows us in the cuts that these men share a common fate: unceasing fear and apprehension, sense of impending disaster, a feeling of hopelessness and utter isolation. One soldier's behavior with the army psychiatrist is so real in his disconnectedness that he seems fake, just a bad actor. That's what battle fatigue produces—bad acting. The victims cannot act, cannot play themselves, which is, of course, the hardest thing to do. The army shrink doesn't think his guys are crazy, but recognizes that outsiders think of their condition as shameful. Forced beyond the limits of human endurance, these changed guys, not the same boys they were when they went in, have reached their breaking point.

I must identify my father, a man under stress, as a psychological casualty. His CO personally aided and abetted his severe stress by prolonging his duty as beach master. In hindsight, we can acknowledge that there probably was a mystery factor operating, but I have no reason to think that my father concealed anything in his application to become an ensign. On the beach, Bill hit the trifecta for intrapsychic conflict: insecurity, sense of duty, obligation to continue. R. R. Grinker, coauthor of *Men under Stress*, cites weak ego, strong sense of duty, anxiety or depression, accusations of malingering, and the fact that they are made to feel that they are cowards as ideal conditions for battle neuroses.

The film catalogues the miraculous cures of some of the men, the army hospital a kind of Lourdes where the holy water of hypnosis, sodium pentathol, occupational therapy, and knowledge of oneself—anger and resentment in deeper parts of the personality—heal the wounded. They play baseball—not my father; they go back to school—my father does. The army has a higher success rate with acute cases of battle neurosis; peacetime neurosis tends to be chronic. In a final send-off, the shrink addresses the problem of anxiety. He says that personal safety stems from childhood safety: children don't grow up well without safety and confidence. When people don't tell their troubles to each other they get anxiety. The soldiers need to find someone they esteem, who makes them feel worthwhile. They need to be fed acceptance. Some part of my father must never have left Tarawa, but he took his troubles to God alone. An African American soldier diagnoses his headaches and crying spells as nostalgia: he means yearning for the past with his sweetheart, with whom he is united at the end of the film.

Nostalgia really means homecoming (*nostos*) + (*algos*), pain, grief, distress. It was considered a disease.

Mom: *In seventh grade I decided to be Joy* [no longer Mercedes] *O'Brien. I was born in Chicago at home. I was the third of four children, not a good place to be in the center, better to be at the beginning or the end. I was born in 1921, so when the stock market fell . . . My father had a lot of money in the stock market and he lost it.*

I went to first grade at St. Lucy's and there were a lot of kids in that room, one nun, big huge room full of kids. Mercedes O'Brien. Aunt Agnes—she was the one that named me Mercedes by the way. I went big duty under the porch, it was muddy, you know it was a mud porch and oh, Aunt Agnes was up in the room and sirens were going, They're coming after you, they're going to get you. A terrible crime, I mean she had me thinking I committed murder.

And then we moved to River Forest, and I went to second grade and third grade at St. Luke's. The confession's in second grade. I can remember running across the street to my mother, this was two, maybe even three years after I went under the porch, and I said I couldn't tell the priest about going big duty under the porch and my mother said, that's not a sin, but Agnes had me paralyzed with fear. I was in first grade and she was at West Suburban Hospital and we lived right around the corner, about a block and a half away. I can remember running home and we prayed for her, we went in the church, the church had deep pillars in the middle of the pews, not everywhere, but I turned around, I was crying about Agnes, and I banged into the pillar, jeez I mean I knocked myself out practically. I was a little kid, you know. That's the first big bang I remember. I went to school to school to school to school. The people that bought the house couldn't pay for it so we went back to Oak Park and they put me at William Buy, which was a public school. On the block there were mean kids I must say, anti-Catholic you know. So I went to fifth and sixth grade at William Buy and they should have left me there, but no, we were going to make our Confirmation so they sent me to seventh grade at St. Lucy's. Then they moved back to River Forest. They said I could go into eighth grade if I went to St. Lucy's from River Forest okay, and so my mother did talk to Miss Schwinn who was the superintendent of schools in River Forest and no, no, no, no I had to go to seventh grade again. I feel bad because I shouldn't a gone. That makes you think you're a loser. Very bad for a kid. And I wasn't dumb. I wasn't brilliant either.

Had my mother been a navy nurse as she had wished, she would, her childhood a catalogue of unsafety, have seen a navy psychiatrist who would have told her that personal safety stems from childhood safety, that children don't grow up well without safety and confidence. He would have advised her that she needed to find someone who would hold her in esteem, who could make her feel worthwhile, who would feed her acceptance.

Saturday April 27, 1974 [fourth entry]

My first project on getting something to do on these days of leisure + time off was to cut the front grass + help my wife pull out an evergreen tree in the front yard. Then we took a ride up to Evanston to visit my daughter Jody, for whom my wife had purchased some clothing at Great Lakes [Naval Base] *recently. We went to the drug store + had milk shakes after which I came home, started watching "The Manchurian Candidate" and promptly fell asleep. So much for this day which promises to fully realize the expectation of another successful weekend.*

W. J. McAuliffe

The Manchurian Candidate puts him promptly to sleep, but he can't be hypnotized. I wonder what he dreams, if he dreams at all. Does he dream what really happened in the South Pacific? Sinatra dreams what really happened in Korea: the Communists, including Laurence Harvey's control-freak mother Angela Lansbury, brainwash Harvey, relieving him of "those uniquely American symptoms of fear and guilt," to kill on command. Sinatra meets Janet Leigh on a train. My father couldn't take a shower for a year after he saw *Psycho*. Janet, resurrected from her shower death, is instantly, irrefutably attracted to Sinatra, a victim of high order post-traumatic stress disorder: he's so disturbed, his hands shaking, he can't light his cigarette. A different kind of controlling female than Angela, she deprograms him and they live happily ever after. Laurence Harvey, on the other hand, who is the Manchurian candidate, dresses up as a priest, shoots his emasculating mother and the Joe McCarthy–clone stepfather, then turns his weapon on himself. My father hated McCarthyism and Nixon, whom he called Tricky Dick. When Roger Marcy, the kid across the street, his nose pressed against the screen door, accuses me of being spoiled rotten—my father calls it Marcyism. Bill with his controlling mother must identify more with the Candidate than with Sinatra. What is it that Bill's mother wants him to kill off? His desire to write plays? He's definitely got a secret inside, but he doesn't know quite what it is—a time bomb ticking away in his brain.

Goodnight, Jim Bob.

Sometimes, when it's very quiet, he can hear the tick.

Part Four

Ourself behind ourself, concealed—
Should startle most—
Assassin hid in our Apartment
Be Horror's least.

C. 1863, EMILY DICKINSON

Saturday May 4, 1974 [fifth entry]

It's pretty difficult to reduce all the events of one week into a single common denominator except to say that last weekend was a complete success. It was a little bit difficult getting back into the harness of everyday living but, bit by bit, + with considerably less confusion than originally anticipated I brought myself up to date on my caseload, + there's just the matter of getting through this weekend successfully. However, I feel just a little depressed + apprehensive about the rest of this day but I know that, with God's help, and the guidance of Doctor Rovner, I can successfully deepen that wedge into the psychological element of my personality. I have got to get through this Saturday without "cracking up." I simply have to do it. Incidentally, I noticed that the last time we visited Jody she seemed a little bit down in the dumps. This diary might serve to be a little life saver in putting my emotions down on paper. Last Tuesday we had a final interview with Maggie + Jim, who were my favorite nurse + orderly at Passavant Hospital. Everything went along smoothly although I did find it a bit difficult answering the probing questions asked me by Maggie + Jim. If I get through this weekend successfully I'll know I have this infamous weekend + holiday syndrome successfully licked. I've the knowledge now of how to do it through the group therapy + assumption of responsibility concepts learned through the efforts of staff + the insight of Doctor Rovner. We took my mother to see Serpico *which was a good movie, but the language was pretty obscene + mother was a little flabbergasted. All in all, good start on a good weekend.*

Adios

Hawaii Pre-Joy

Tennessee Williams's *The Glass Menagerie* opens in Chicago on December 26, 1944, and runs while Bill is stateside but not yet discharged.

Laurette Taylor finds the play she has been waiting for and Bill sees it. An indelible image of excellence, her miraculous performance in this dream/nightmare of loss, loss, loss, takes up permanent residence in his mind. It was for him one of those life-changing moments in the theater—a moment of intensity more real than so-called real life, and one of the few things he told me about his past that actually happened. The hero joins the merchant seamen, refuses responsibility for his mother and crippled sister, and embraces his vocation as a writer. One night in the theater can flip the switch, convince Bill that theater is what he needs in order to live. A model, a possibility that he might be good enough. The war ends and he returns to the South Pacific in 1950 for graduate study in English and theater at the University of Hawaii. I learn this from his obituary. You'd think he might have told me himself. Bill never talks about his having wanted to write plays. In his despair as a writer, he never attends a professional production from the time I am born until his death—*The Glass Menagerie* perhaps the last performance he ever saw. He never mentions any other.

On the blind, I write to the current chair of the Department of Theatre and Dance of the University of Hawaii at Manoa to find out what kinds of courses my father may have taken there. He writes back suggesting he'll go to the bound volumes of the playwriting classes taught by Willard Wilson, part of the postwar explosion of writing programs, to try to find a copy of my father's script. Aloha.

Two weeks later he will send me two one-act plays written by my father, from a bound volume in the library there, with an introduction by the professor at that time, including his notes on my father's plays. I am stunned to receive these early, usually autobiographical plays—a window on his soul.

Jody:

Your father wrote two one-act plays here in Fall 1950 in the English Department Playwriting class of Prof. Willard Wilson. Wilson was a pioneer in the development of playwriting in the state. The plays are in volume 6 of 'College Plays', call. no. PN 6120.C6H39 (an unpaginated but bound typescript). I'm not sure what involvement your father may have had in the Dept of Drama and Theatre when it separated away from English in 1952, or even if he was still here then, but it appears that neither of his plays was actually produced by the

University Theatre Guild, later renamed University Theatre Group. I have copies of a very interesting Preface by Wilson in which he comments on both of the plays, and I could send you this and xeroxed copies of the plays if you like.

Both plays have a sophisticated sense of technical and scenic theatre.

The first, 'Strata,' deals with three levels of society through separate sets at different heights. Down-and-outs, middle class and aristocrats play out a Morality in which Death finally claims the dead-beat man and the aristocratic wife. The other play is rather like a comic 'No Exit' in which a ghost couple on a Pacific island, English aristocrat and Vassar woman, argue and create their hell five years after they have drowned, with comic tension provided by a dead butler, in jeans and butler jacket, and an American survivor of another wreck. Its action is 'circular' but the dialogue is tart and effective.

Hope this is helpful.

Aloha,
W. Dennis Carroll

Sophisticated. Tart and effective. I'm in shock. The five years between the end of the war and Bill's return to Hawaii to study is lost to me, yet two of his plays arrive, in print no less. The biggest shocker—they're good! I'm developing an image of the writer writing: a graduate student in Honolulu, Bill lives in an apartment with his older brother Jack and Mary Jane, Jack's new bride, types into the wee hours of the night, sending me coded messages—images, gestures, ideas—from the other side. My brother tells me that Bill was a communications officer, and well-versed in semaphore and Morse code, among other means. He says, When I was learning Morse for Boy Scouts, Bill claimed to have forgotten, but he still knew it—probably just didn't want to think about it.

The plays reveal his sensibility, his consciousness, his taste, his obsessions: the arbitrariness of death, the obliviousness of aristocratic and business classes to suffering. After a promising start of two semesters and one summer session, he drops out before he finishes his master's. Returns to Oak Park and adapts plays for the Edmund players, a community theater group based in the church he grew up in. Takes a job in business, of all things. Something happened.

When my brother stays with Uncle Jack and Aunt Mary Jane in

Hawaii half a century later, he plays his bass till the wee hours of the morning. Mary Jane tells him he reminds her of our father, the way he typed all night. Joy said it was awkward for Bill, living with the newlyweds, but that couldn't have been why he dropped out. Professor Wilson's preface mentions housing difficulties in Honolulu, but my brother says, if Bill had wanted it badly enough, he could have found another place to live. Maybe it was the writing. Maybe it was the vultures, already beginning to gather.

Wilson: *The really frightening little sketch*, Strata, *also by Mr. McAuliffe, is a vicious satire on the constant sociological and biological scramble for the top of the heap. The 'simultaneous staging' and symbolism have possibilities that are* not fully realized *because they are* not consistently exploited *throughout the play; but the ideas are* worthy of more experiment and elaboration *in the one-act form.*

Wilson goes on to suggest that Bill, like many young writers, concentrates on dialogue and fails to visualize clearly other dramatic possibilities. He is not certain just what the author is trying to tell us. *It is unfortunate in a way, also, that the author was not able to work into the fibre of the play some of the element of compassion, without which the spectacle of debased men and women is more often nauseating than dramatically moving. The touch of the absolving priest on the lower level is hardly adequate to sound the note clearly.*

If only Bill had focused on the positive: really frightening, vicious satire. And on the constructive: possibilities that need to be realized and exploited throughout, ideas that are worthy of more experiment and elaboration, the need to refine what he's trying to say. Maybe he would have continued to write plays—momentary stays against confusion. He might have developed his craft, and found a different way to live. Was it a case of his having judged himself not good enough? Or was the gorilla with the gun—a darkness there behind Bill's eyes, visible to my brother in the 1953 wedding portrait—commandeering a new room in Bill's brain, preventing him from tackling the challenge of the craft of writing, preventing a necessary consistency?

Strata begins with thunder, lightning, and a terrifying scream, what he must have experienced on a regular basis in the tropics during the war. Their actions punctuated by thunder, two figures, a derelict and another man, struggle to the death—an event that makes no difference to the aristocrats and the business class in the world of the play, oblivious as they are to the suffering of the derelict below. It almost feels like a governing metaphor for my father's life to come. The smartly refined upper-class wife, Eloise, thinks she hears a scream from the rotting, verminous alleys down below, a hell from which she's exquisitely happy to be infinitely removed. When the Man sticks the Derelict with a knife, leaving him to suffer and writhe fitfully throughout the play, Eloise is suddenly dreadfully disrupted by what goes on in the street. Self-medicated with cigarettes and cocktails, she's disrupted by her memory, the memory customarily disciplined by her husband. With a powerfully physical stage direction, Bill describes a repulsive-looking cripple dragging himself onstage and swarming all over the dying man. His arms work in quick jerky movements as he ferrets out various objects from the man's pockets, stows them within his own rags, then drags himself hideously off. In war, soldiers have to prey on the dead in order to survive. At that very moment, the upper-class woman staggers and clutches at her chest in sympathy with the dying man on the street below: third time this week, she says, the syndrome progressive. Beach Boss Bill, in sympathy with the marines being slaughtered before his eyes, staggers and clutches at his chest. Eloise's husband George tells her to exercise her will against what she calls a wall of pain: "I suggest you exercise your will more strongly against these neurotic spasms." His method of keeping what Strindberg called "the dirt of life" at a distance is ominously close to what Dr. Rovner will tell Bill twenty-four years later about his spells: exercise your will against these spasms. In the play, neither the social-climbing businessman nor the aristocrat has time for pain, aches, or getting sick.

In his book with Dr. Sandra Aamodt, *Welcome to Your Brain*, Dr. Sam Wang says: "Making choices and decisions, making plans to act, and carrying out those plans call upon a resource that can be depleted." Willpower is finite; nobody knows why. It is reduced under conditions of stress. One effort of will interferes with a second. You can exercise your willpower—boot camp's a good place for this—but if there's a gorilla in your anterior cingulated cortex, your attention and decision making are impaired. Bill professes to believe in the power of the mind: one of the books that fell on our heads that I never see him reading is *The Power of Positive Thinking* by Norman Vincent Peale, originally published in 1952. Strengthening your brain will physically change your brain. Now I can recognize the true strength of Bill's willpower, how stubbornly he fought to hold it together against that gorilla, a force much stronger than his will.

George meets Eloise's complaint of pain and not feeling at all well with, "A simple exercise of willpower is all that is necessary to destroy this absurd hallucination of yours, Eloise!" The xenophobia of the crass business couple causes Eloise to clutch at her chest, but she doesn't understand why. Bill, who regularly derided materialism and the glorification of the Almighty Dollar, uses the play to rail against the aristocratic bastards, the bourgeoisie who love only money, and the swinishness of the people on the street. My father's loathing of American business comes through vividly in this scathing satire of the American businessman, with his anti-immigration stance and aspiration to join the ruling class in its utter lack of humanity. The touch of the absolving priest on the lower level is not meant to sound a clear note of compassion, but rather suggests the emptiness of religion. After he gives last rites to the stabbing victim, Eloise staggers into the living room and crumples to the floor. They all think she's asleep instead of dead. At that point George and the business couple finally see the stabbing victim on the street below. It's the first they've seen of death and its horror, but the Beach Boss saw Death fall on all, indifferently, every day. There are no strata: we're just plain dead. The aristocrat and the businessman declare themselves unkillable, even as they carry out Eloise's dead body. They've learned nothing. The businessman's final line is a xenophobic war cry: "I've got no use for foreigners! I'm a businessman! A one hunnerd per cent American businessman!!" A masked figure of Death appears at the end of the play. He warns against writing: "What phrases are you twisting and turning, trying to define the undefinable. I'll be back! My memory is a sea of faces; pale flames lighting the wilderness of time!" The no-doubt-unconscious echo of Ezra Pound's *In a Station of the Metro* suggests that maybe Bill wasn't a playwright, but rather a lyric poet:

> The apparition of these faces in the crowd;
> Petals on a wet, black bough.

Professor Wilson's Preface comments on Bill's second play, *Draw One for Tea*: *The thing that makes Sartre's play* [No Exit] *and Mr. McAuliffe's theoretically so much more horrible than* Hedda [Gabler] *is that whereas that bored lady could and did escape by suicide, these 20th Century people are already dead, and literally have no exit from their torment.* Bill's *Draw One for Tea*, set on a desert island/country club of a hell, bears a striking resemblance to Strindberg's *Dance of Death*. Lady Phipps, desperate to attract Lord Phipps, both drowned five years ago, struggles vainly to ignite her love life with her dead husband. Lord Phipps cares only about playing cards—the great McAuliffe obsession. Stuck with a frustrating game of solitaire, because Lady Phipps has hidden an ace, he longs for a third to join in a game of his beloved bridge—"mental hand to hand combat" with "no room for class distinction." Lady Phipps, a hopeless romantic lusting for action, sees everything around her as a painful reminder of what's missing from her life. The real hell is death in life. For Bill, then, is hell the inability to escape from bores? No wonder he finds making small talk so difficult.

My father always lamented that he couldn't do small talk. His torticollis may have caused him to be anxious in certain social situations. At a barbecue in Downers Grove with my mother, shortly after they were married, he drank martinis, went upstairs, and fell asleep or passed out. Joy was embarrassed and so was Bill. After that he stopped drinking altogether. By combining phenobarbital with alcohol—two depressants—he became drunk more easily. That particular combo makes alcohol burn off very slowly. I never saw him touch alcohol. He told me he didn't drink because of all the medications. My brother tells me that he started bidding wildly at bridge—another sign of his mental deterioration—and our mother didn't want to play with him anymore. She found it humiliating. Betting strictly within your means was that important.

In *Draw One for Tea*, Bill's beach, the primal scene of his metamorphosis, is "millions of young boy and girl grains of sand—snuggling up close together and kissing the daylight out of each other! And it keeps right on going on and on!" Lady Phipps: "In the last analysis that's all everything is—one everlasting kiss!" I had no idea that my father was such a romantic, such a sensualist. After a still-living, breathing male body washes up on the beach, Lord Phipps persuades the newcomer to choose a hand of bridge over a dance with his wife.

Lady Phipps loses. The waves expire on the lonely beach, their last gasp dying in each other's arms.

Somehow fishing that hole of a navy in the South Pacific, Bill gets hooked in the branches. The ocean turns out to be a swamp. After the summer of '51, Bill realizes he doesn't want to be in Hawaii anymore, the water deepening. It's up to his armpits. Getting a master's in playwriting proves impossible. The writing turns tragic and graduate school becomes a tragic adventure. He does not want to stay. He has written two plays, but the University Theatre Guild does not produce his work. Somewhere in there he writes the infamous *Strange Music*, the play lost in the attic, and heads back to narrow-minded Oak Park. The days of fishing the swamp—bare banks and patchy sun, impossible to walk through—are coming. They will bring him low. He won't be able to go back. By never talking about it to his children, he will try to avoid looking back.

With my father's death certificate and my birth certificate, I succeed in obtaining his transcript.

Fall 1950	
Playwriting	B
Shakespeare	C
Acting	C
Aesthetics of Theatre	C
Spring 1951	
Fiction Writing	B
Types of Drama	B
Shakespeare Tragedies	C
History of Theatre	B
Summer 1951	
Acting	B
Literature of Pacific	C

Teaching, as I do, in an era of grade inflation, I have to say I'm surprised by the grades, as if he's my child and I think he should be doing better, even if he gets a B in both writing courses, and his acting improves. The tale told by the transcript does not include his reason for quitting. But I know the reason, don't I? Sometimes, when it's very quiet, I can hear the tick.

The Saturday Night Swindle

Joy: *They were looking for nurses in Hawaii and I said jeez I think I'll go. I was thinking about going to Hawaii. The funny thing was, Bill McAuliffe was in Hawaii at that time. I didn't know him, but I did know Jack McAuliffe and he was in Hawaii, he lived there. I knew him from Peggy* [my mother's older sister], *she double dated with Jack McAuliffe and Johnny O, who was his roommate at Notre Dame. She said Jack McAuliffe thought he was God Almighty. But that doesn't matter, thing is I knew Jack McAuliffe was from Oak Park, I might have gotten in touch with him, and Bill McAuliffe was going to University of Hawaii then. I don't know what he was doing. He was a terrible writer I hate to tell you, he was bum, not good at all, not good at all. I read one thing he wrote, that didn't get a . . . he had submitted it and it wasn't good, it was a short story.*

Not once but five times he's no good. My brother finds this extremely disturbing. My mother acted in a community theater production of *The Man Who Came to Dinner* before I was born, but had no discernible urge to get back on the boards. Whether she told my father she thought he was a bad writer, I'll never know. Never any good at filtering her language, had she opened her mouth on the subject, the unlaundered words would have tumbled right out. When I had the opportunity to ask her if she told him, the question failed to occur to me. Now it's too late. I certainly never heard her encourage him to write. Sensitive as he was to atmosphere, he must have known what she thought of him as a writer, whether she said anything or not.

Joy: *And Ralph O* [her cousin] *knew Bill McAuliffe from St. Edmund's, he was in the Edmund Players or something, writing, writing, writing plays after college, after the navy, 1951. This thing that he wrote though, the story that he had submitted was nothing, you know. He started writing plays, it wasn't he was writing plays, he was fixing plays that were made to put on the shows. Ralph O was eight years younger than I was but he was in the Edmund Players. Anyway, Ralph brought—they came over to my house, Bill thought I was Ralph's date and the other girl was his date. He told me that later, but that night he went home to Aunt Josie and said I met the girl I'm going to marry. I didn't know that. I can't imagine why, poor devil.*

Poor devil. Little did she know their meeting—the ultimate Saturday night swindle, breakdown, blind-as-a-bat first date—though far from a bus accident, was surely an accident looking for a place to happen. As a junior in college, when I tell my mother that my female roommate and I will have a male roommate, she tries to warn me off of it: "You never know, he might come out of the closet with an axe." Metaphorically speaking, that's what my father did to her. He came out of the closet with the behavioral equivalent of an axe, fulfilling her worst nightmare: that she, a nurse, would be condemned to care for an invalid in her own home for the majority of her married life. No wonder *The Fugitive* was her favorite show.

Saturday May 11 [sixth entry]

Well this last weekend almost proved to be a disaster. I had a seizure down at work Thursday afternoon, + Joy had to come down + pick me up at the office. I am just now pulling out of this thing + I think that with the help of God I can make this weekend a little better + easier. We went down to see Dr. Rovner today + he also stated that I should pull myself together + not destroy Joy + the kids because of my mental insecurity. We had a nice dinner at Otto's today + I enjoyed it very much. However, I am going to have to exert more self control from now on. This is Saturday nite + I think I have myself under control now. I played some of my Oscar Peterson records tonite but will have to do something tomorrow. If we don't have dinner with Brien tomorrow I'll have to do something on my own or with Joy. I drove the car for the first time in over a year today + that did a lot toward restoring my confidence in myself. I hope I'll be able to go to church tomorrow + we'll have a nice weekend maybe dinner with all the kids. Well, I'm very tired now + think maybe I'll be better tomorrow.

WJMcAuliffe

Joy: *Back up here a little bit. I was working at the telephone company right after high school, and Roslyn and Herb Simon came over. Herb Simon wanted to introduce me to Ralph Ianni. He went to the University of Kentucky then; he played football at Oak Park River Forest High School. I didn't know him at all, never saw him. Then we dated and everything, you know, and the next year he went in the navy air corps. We went down to Armstrongs' and Mr. Armstrong had been in the navy and he was talking to Ralph, and anyway Ralph went into the navy air corps. And one thing that I did—he wanted me to come down to Florida to Pensacola to get his wings and I was going I thought, and I went and got suitcases, but I didn't have clothes right or anything. I was ignorant, a dumb kid, and anyway I changed my mind. I didn't go. It was a terrible thing—he wanting and needing to have somebody go down there when he picked up his wings. Just didn't go. I don't know why I didn't go, lazy, just didn't do it, should'a done it. It was a cruel thing to leave him with nobody there. I've thought of that and I thought oh boy, what a dumb thing. I was nineteen. When he came home, one thing—we went to see* Oklahoma. *I remember that. That was very nice. He was in the navy then and he sent me money to buy a ring and I had it at that time. It was $300 and that was a lot of money, it'd be like a $1000 now and I put it in the bank. Well anyway he was killed then. And uh.*

No he wasn't killed, he was lost in action. That was 1943. Then I went into the nurse corps. That's when I went in. I really wanted . . . see I would have been in the war. If I'd gone in '40 I probably would have been in the war cause I was wantin' to be a navy nurse, you know. By the time I got out it was 1947 and the war was over.

He was never found, they never found him.

I don't want to talk anymore.

So my mother did, in fact, have a first love whom she lost tragically in the war. In a snapshot they're standing in front of a tree and Ralph is himself a tree—handsome, healthy, and strong, two heads taller than my mother, who is a stand-in for Rosalind Russell. In high school she took French and Latin because she wanted to be a nurse. She applied to St. Francis in Evanston, which is a good hospital, and her aunt lived a few blocks away. Her father didn't send the application. Her parents decided that she'd change her mind so they didn't send it. June came along and she thought, gee, they haven't called me. Her parents never sent it; then they sent it too late and she didn't get in. She asked, Why haven't they called? Like characters in one of those Irish plays where the controlling parent traps the child by hiding the letter promising romance and escape—a shot at a different life—they told her, We never sent it. I, of Irish heritage and a theater director, can't stand those Irish plays. They make me want to scream. Then the cadet nurse corps was looking for nurses and the government paid. See, her parents were short of money, too. Had she gone to St. Francis she would have had to pay money. The cadet corps paid for uniforms and everything. She, Mercedes O'Brien, was in a room with Phil O'Brien (her sister), Joan O'Brien, and Loretta Finlay; so it was O'Brien, O'Brien, O'Brien, and Finlay on the door and they thought that was hilarious.

Joy: *My parents didn't have a lot of money, and I tell you we didn't have any jobs at all and I'm thinking to myself jeez what could we have done to make some money to give to my dad, you know. When he was at the bank forty-three years, he retired, but he died soon after that. He had a heart attack at home. When he was a kid, he was very good in grammar school, long jump, and they found out he had some kind of a heart—whatever I had he had—so he stopped the long jump. He was always a moderate man, moderate everything, he worked hard you know, he had all these houses—the one in Oak Park, and the one on Wilcox, and the one in River Forest. He was real estate poor, and he had to pay taxes and he wasn't getting any money for 'em. I'm thinking to myself wasn't it a shame that we couldn't have done something to make some money. And then that was a dumb trick, too, when I graduated, instead of working at the hospital or something I worked for the Armstrongs, in the next block, and for three years took care of their invalid grandma. Just easy, I guess, foolish, dumb. I was making $70 a week, that was good pay, and I wasn't using my talent. I learned a lot though, about cleaning a house. For three years.*

Then she met Bill. Can it be that my mother thought his head on his ear suited him marvelously, that she thought him pretty? He is very pretty in the pre-torticollian navy picture with his older brother Jack in the foreground. Bill looks straight at the camera, resolute. I think I know that he didn't think he was pretty, post-torticollis, though he never mentioned it.

> My poor body is shortened
> And I have my head on my ear
> But it suits me marvelously
> And among the torticollis
> I pass for one of the prettiest (Scarron, 1610–1660)

The French *tort*: wrong, evil. The OED defines wryness as the fact or condition of being distorted. Wry also means to conceal or hide.

It was the French poet Scarron who first used the present form torticollis. A deformity, if it is that—an ugliness or depravity hard to miss—torticollis has been known as long as people have had the capacity to stare at each other. Plutarch notes in his *Lives*, Alexander the Great's "manner of holding his neck hanging down towards the left side." Alexander was known for his physical beauty. Is it true that lateral inclination of the head is favored by saints and other distinguished people? I drag out *The Day Book of the Saints* to check out this observation, and I do see a torticollian bent in the paintings of medieval saints, especially in the depictions of those in the process of having a vision, and those in the process of turning their awestruck, grace-filled gazes respectfully from Heaven.

My father, the alleged (favorite word because it means so-called, declared, but without proof) Apocalyptic Horseman, Admiral in the Japanese Navy, and leader of a long planned but never executed safari to Basutoland, was wry long before and long after his neck twisted and turned. In the medieval understanding of wryness, his wry-neck is an expression of his particular sense of humor: our bodies allegories of our personalities. He turns his head and faces to the right, alters his course, stops writing until he begins what he hopes is a life-saving diary during what he knows is the last year of his life.

Bill takes Joy down to Ricket's on Rush Street—it was in November or October, very dramatic, very romantic—and asks her to marry him. They were talking about getting married at Thanksgiving, and why they didn't get married on Thanksgiving, she doesn't know. So they got married on January 15. It was snowing, too—not snowing, slushy—and they had the breakfast at the Oak Park Arms. They went to the Edgewater Beach Hotel right on Lake Michigan. It was very nice. They went downtown to see a pianist, William . . . William . . . He was a very good pianist, at the Blackstone or something. She did not share my father's passion for jazz. They had lunch with one of his friends from work. He was working at the rubber company, U.S. Something, U.S. Rubber. It was '53.

Saturday May 18, 1974 [seventh entry]

Well, today marks the beginning of a new era in my life. I mean that this is the first Saturday in about the last six years that I have not cracked up. I believe the success of this day is due mostly to God, + second mostly, to the success of Doctor Rovner's psychological insight into my trouble. I feel so good too that once again I'm able to drive the car. It makes a big difference. Today we drove up to Dr. Rovner's office, then, on to have lunch with Jody. I have a feeling now, an overpowering confidence that I can break this disastrous pattern for good + all. It has to do with having something to do in my off days. Jody was glad to see us. Hope I can continue the good work. Till next week. Adios WJMcAuliffe

On this business of driving the car: my mother, an incorrigible back-seat driver, could barely sit in a car with anybody else behind the wheel, without putting the imaginary pedal to the metal in the midst of her running corrective commentary. Her desire to always be driving restricted my father to life as a perpetual passenger, dependent on her and lacking in confidence.

Does Joy marry Bill despite or because of his torticollis? On the face of it, as it were, his is a head that is off its center, loose, not well connected to his body, free floating, a head he cannot control or keep still, a head that is unstable. Erving Goffman might suggest that his torticollis was a disguise put on him without his consent or knowledge, as in a fairy tale, that it confused him as to his own identity. He couldn't recognize himself in the mirror anymore, but my mother carried none of the baggage that this was a sign of weakness. She, street smart but with an acute sense of her own self as not book smart, after barely surviving attendance at nine different grammar schools, must have found herself reflected in some way in torticollitic Bill, even though it was Bill who fell hard on the blinded date. Before surgery he was a broad-shouldered athletic guy who happened to have torticollis. Not seeing his invalid potential, she subconsciously chose to face her worst fear. Seemingly inevitably, she brought the thing she feared most crashing down on all of our heads. Sally, the nine-year-old girl, loved him too, despite or because of his affliction. Maybe torticollis, like tuberculosis, suggests heightened sensitivity—he was sensitive. I loved him, more than I loved my mother while he was alive. I came to love my mother much later, in my thirties. I didn't care about his hidden/fantasy past, a blank slate for me to write on: he was good to me. My mother spilled that he had frequented prostitutes before he knew her, because, he said, he could talk to them. When I tell my mother that I like my father better than her—maybe I am six years old—she tells me that he doesn't really like to take care of us when she goes bowling on Wednesdays: it makes him afraid.

Saturday May 25 [eighth entry]

I am writing this on Sunday May 26 instead of Saturday May 25. Anyway, this probably will qualify as one of the lousiest weekends in history. Yesterday the paper was a little bit late in arriving so that threw me off + now today being allegedly Sunday I've really screwed up everything. So that's it + I'll just have to do a little bit better tomorrow.

Adios,
WJMcAuliffe

The young couple—with their baby son and first child, Brien, in tow—buys a house in Westchester.

Joy: *We were lookin' at houses and Mr. McAuliffe, Bill's father, said this is the one. It was twenty-one, which was low, which was good. It wasn't beyond us. We were lucky, he said, you get that. So we did, and he—it was auctioned the next day, but he got it. He fixed it so we got it for twenty-one. Mr. McAuliffe paid cash, I think. Then Bill's brother Jack told Brien that Mr. McAuliffe bought the house, and I didn't think he should do that, and I wrote a letter.*

I had money. We paid Mr. McAuliffe back. We had just sold my parents' house in River Forest and split it up four ways. I had the $5000, but that isn't the way the story went. I wrote Jack a letter and I said I didn't think you should do that. Anyway, I don't care who bought the house, you don't tell a kid that the grandfather bought the house. To me—I didn't think that was right.

And another thing Bill insisted on doing was getting a mortgage insurance. We didn't know it was paid for because we weren't told. We were paying for the house to George Baker actually, but it was to Mr. McAuliffe because he used that name. He did this all secretively, legal-wise I suppose.

Mr. McAuliffe wasn't poor, see. Mary wasted it all. Mrs. McAuliffe died a pauper and Mary was a pauper, except she owned two pianos and paid twenty dollars a month at least to store them. I'm just saying, he gave us money, but he gave them money, too. We couldn't have bought it, or we wouldn't have gotten it at the time. We couldn't have gotten this house if it weren't paid cash, and they had to go to the bank to get the money.

We moved in in July and you were born in November.

Standing on End

The doctors' voices seem to come from the next room. He cannot really feel anything, but he hears them cutting the ropes that hold the mast of his body in its twisted shape.

"You've got a beautiful back. I am looking forward to working on that."

"But will it cure me?"

He slaps him on the back.

"We'll sure take a crack at it, eh boy?"

He sees the world differently since the war.

After a while he slips into some bluer zone.

"I'm going to have another baby," my mother tells him.

"How is that possible?"

"Don't you remember?"

"Yes, but I thought since you were nursing—"

"I guess that's just a story."

"It's going to be hard. I'm not working and I have to have the surgery. They tell me it's a long recovery period."

"What do you want me to do?"

"I'm happy, really. Just scared."

"Me too."

The first time he wakes up he thinks he is dying. His neck is killing him. He opens the window and feels the cold air stinging his naked body. He thinks he's going to fall out. Then he feels the light touch of fingers like spider webs weaving over his hands and feet. The sensation is not unpleasant. The golden powder from his wings sticks on their fingers. They cannot get it off. It starts pouring out of him. They cannot stop its flow. He feels it collect in his throat so that he almost suffocates. He cannot seem to swallow. The whole place in there is airless. A hollow forms and he imagines his baby molded from the powder of his wings, nurtured in his twisted neck, set free by the cutting of the nerves.

I am born. He tries to kill himself by jumping out the window of the hospital and has to be restrained. Without language there is no point in going on.

He wakes up with a mouthful of sand. His hands and feet are restrained. He remembers the window. It was the not being able to speak that made him do it and he couldn't swallow.

My mother goes to visit him.

"Why did you do it? You shouldn't have."

He still can't talk. He doesn't really know what he did, he was so doped up. He half smiles.

"They wouldn't let me bring the baby, but she is beautiful."

He mouths, what color is her hair?

She cannot understand him so he tries again.

"It's red, like yours. Standing on end."

He knows what that's like. She holds him until it is time for her to go.

He can speak a little now so they remove the restraints. They know he won't try to hurt himself again. He reads *The Tempest* until he cannot keep his eyes open. When he closes his eyes he hears Benny Goodman and moves his fingers on his chest along with the music. When it comes time for his solo he can't move. Benny goes on without him.

His wife takes him home from the hospital. His little boy is with her. He is dressed in a sailor suit which makes him laugh, but in secret. He still hasn't seen the girl except in his head. He always thinks of me in a Red Flyer wearing a white dress. My hair matches the color of the wagon. For my wedding he will suggest that I ride down the aisle in the wagon. That will make me smile when I'm older.

His wife holds me up to show him.

"See, she looks just like you."

He has never seen anything so strange.

His wife goes back to work while he recovers. Wednesday is her bowling night. His little boy and he watch TV while his little girl sleeps. But I don't sleep. I cry. He only cries in his dreams. It will take me a while to learn how to do that.

He tells his boy his favorite one about how he was a commander in the Japanese navy.

The boy can't understand him, but he laughs in color. I am screaming. It starts as a shiver at his nerve endings. He turns up the TV, but I pierce through that.

"Pajamas on!"

His little son jumps to attention.

"Ready, march. One, two, three, four. One, two, three, four."

His little legs goose-step down the hall. He sits very still for a minute, counting to sixty. I wail.

Finally he gets up and walks down the hallway. He closes my door and goes to his son's room. Good boy, he's all tucked in. Turns his bright eyes up to his father.

"You're a good soldier."

His son smiles and he kisses his eyes. Put out the light.

And then put out the light. He hovers outside my door. I am really screaming now. He thinks his skull is cracking and what's the matter with me anyway?

Inside the room he paces in the darkness, talking, trying to make me stop. The only rhyme he can think of is "ain't no use in going home, Jody's got your girl and gone; ain't no use in looking back"—he reaches into the crib to pick me up. Instead he grabs my arm and rips it hard like a rope start on an outboard engine. I stop. He switches the light on and I'm not dead, just quiet. I'm gonna get me a three-day pass, gonna go home whoop Jody's ass.

He has to take me to the emergency room. He's holding me as he opens his son's door. With one free hand he picks the boy up and runs out of the house. Our lives are in his hands now.

Saturday 6-1-74 [ninth entry]

This has been one of characteristically the most disastrous weekends in my life. I had one of my sudden spells down at work the other day; I pushed the panic button + Joy had to come down + pick me up. Then I apparently threw a real fit here because Joy hit me in the ribs with a terrific wallop + I'm certain one or more of my ribs on the left side is broken. Moreover, everyone has to line up against me; nobody is ever for me. Whatever bad happens it's all my fault always mine. Nobody will ever lift a finger in my defense. [I notice my brother made the same complaint: Mom just stood by and there was no one there to defend me. There was no one to defend me ever.] *Anyway Dr. Rovner told me that I must improve psychologically in my own mind. It is going to be a long hard struggle. I know that the going will not be easy, or else I will drive everyone else around me crazy. For the moment then Adios*

WJMcAuliffe

Saturdays are bleeding into Sundays and sometimes he can't get through the week at work. If he makes it past Wednesday he's feeling lucky. Up to four packs of Viceroys a day. He hides two inside his suit coat so Joy won't find out. She drives him to the bus that takes him to the "L" that takes him downtown to the place where he works. Sometimes, his friend Tom, his best friend at work, drives him. Tom is simple and good, a dese, dem, dose kind of guy. They plan to go out to lunch, but a client of Tom's appears and Bill is on his own. After the fact, Bill will hear that the client used inappropriate language and Tom told him his mother wouldn't like to hear him talk that way. The client didn't like that. Then something happened. After lunch, Bill waits for the elevator to return to the office. The doors open and there on a gurney lies poor Tom's body. Bill sees his crushed skull and for a split second he is back on the beach. This time, it's Jack who gets the panicked phone call to rescue Bill. By the time Jack makes it down to the office, Bill has returned to himself. Jack finds him sitting in his boss's office talking calmly with him. His boss tells Jack, "We could sure use some more Bill McAuliffes around here."

Saturday 6-8-74 [tenth entry]

Well, this is one weekend that has simply got to work out for the salvation of the sanity of everyone in the family, particularly Joy, who is having her problems + poor Jack, who I'm certain would be completely nuts if he has to put up with my indigenous behavior from now until I die. As Dr. Rovner put it, the major portion of my problem is psychological. I really have to work at this otherwise I'm doomed. Last weekend I couldn't even concentrate on a game of cards with Mary

+ Mother. Jack is through school now + yesterday pulled a hamstring muscle in his leg, but, fortunately is feeling much better today. Jody will be home Monday for the summer, + I am taking my summer vacation 8-16-74 through Labor Day which should make everyone reasonably happy. It's approaching critical time of the day now when I either start pulling myself together or not. I think I can do it today now because the major part of the battle is over. The Daily News has arrived, now I have an appointment with Dr. Rovner at 11: 45 today.

Adios

Bill reads *The Fire Next Time* (1963) and *Black Like Me* (1961); he joins the NAACP. I sneak his books from his bedside table and sample them. When I find, "Hey, shithead," in *Black Like Me*, I think I'm pretty cool and so's my dad. He fought the fight every day down at the office, which he called "the salt mine," counseling the drunks, prostitutes, and other unhappy individuals. Anti-capitalist, egalitarian, deeply humane Bill—a rebel and I didn't even know it—never lost his conscience.

Saturday June 22, 1974 [twelfth entry]

Well, at least I can say that this has been one of my more successful weekends. With one notable exception—last week I had pains in my chest, and, I, naturally assumed immediately, I was scared stiff that a heart attack was imminent; so they called the Fire Dept ambulance + rushed me over to Mercy Hospital by which time, of course, the pains had completely disappeared. I felt such a complete ass, being rushed to the hospital for nothing, not even oxygen. This time I thought for sure, I had really blown it. But eventually I did recover although my desk is still in turmoil + I'm not certain whether I'll ever be able to straighten it out again. However, I have managed to push through a few hires. Anyway, Saturday + Sunday were ok. The trouble is that these attacks or spells come on me without warning and once they start they cannot be stopped. They just have to run their devastating course destroying everyone in their path. I have sometimes felt so depressed that I could commit suicide except I just haven't got the "guts." My twice weekly alcoholics anonymous meetings have been extremely successful to start. Four or five are really "making it" one day at a time. Of course there are those who are still drinking but they are coming to the meetings regularly + not just for the carfare. I am deeply interested in helping these alcoholics who are trying to help themselves. I feel an affinity for these men + women because I can really relate to them. Also I am extremely grateful for the help I am getting from Walter S. My kids all love me except when I'm in one of those spells, which are always hell for me. Anyway I've had a good weekend so far, + more than that no man can expect.

WJMcAuliffe

Usually AA meetings are run by members of AA, members with at least a year of sobriety, but the types of cases he dealt with as a vocational counselor at the Department of Labor required him to hold and run meetings so that he could find jobs for the recovering alcoholics. He relates to them because his spells are like benders, lost weekends, dry blackouts. He blames himself, with the neurologist's help, for the so-called spells—what the doctor regards as lapses in willpower as opposed to dementia. He identifies with alcoholics because he suffers from what feels like a spiritual malaise from which he can never be cured; he can only be recovering, for as long he lives. If he truly was in AA I never knew it, and neither did my mother or brothers. Maybe he told the priest or the Virgin Mary to whom he prayed daily, rosary in hand, when he came home from work and lay down before dinner, seeking through prayer and meditation to improve his conscious contact with God, praying only for knowledge of His will for him and the power to carry it out—the eleventh step.

He did receive an exorcism once, a highly secretive affair. I was not invited—not to my cousins' funeral and not to my father's exorcism. My mother, a member of the holy-rolling Third Order of Franciscans, arranged for it to be conducted at the Franciscan seminary near our house, a magical place where we went for midnight masses at Christmas; the relics of a saint who looked like a shriveled midget lay in the chapel in a tiny glass coffin. We played hide-and-seek amid the cherry velvet curtains. It was scary and beautiful, like when I played the angel in church, wearing wings, kissing red rose petals, and dropping them to the ground as I walked up the aisle during the Stations of the Cross. In the name of God, they tried to drive out the demon that must have been infesting my father, making him a victim and instrument of his malice. Exorcism, in Bill's case, did not work, maybe because there was no evil spirit inside of him—or because what was inside was more powerful than the exorcist.

Saturday June 29, 1974 [thirteenth entry]

I guess this weekend must qualify as one of the worst, the crappiest weekend in history. For some reason I am so confused now that I don't know where to turn. Everyone seems against me as usual. I don't know why or what went wrong.

Everything I touch I destroy. I many times think that it would be best for everyone if I were dead. But then I recall how my own soul would rot in eternity if I played God + took my own life. I will have to keep it up to the end—destroy, destroy, destroy. When this thing happens to me it comes on with no warning; + there seems to be no controlling it once it starts. No matter what I try it just doesn't work. I try + try + try but all I hear is shut up, shut up, shut up. I'm up a real tree now + they are all against me. So much for that.

WJMcAuliffe

The day my parents drive me to college in Evanston, I'm not sure if we still have the GTO my older brother talked my mother into buying for the family car—the one I drive to Notre Dame to visit my cousin, at speeds around one hundred miles an hour, when I'm still in high school. In my family, on my mother's side, we are the opposite of risk averse. I become a freshman at Northwestern without visiting any colleges before enrolling. I don't want to go there and I don't want to go into theater. I have it in my head that I want to be a lawyer like my grandfather and uncle. Though I always think I am making my own choices, I am, in actuality, driven by the invisible, unintentional will—there is such an oxymoronic thing—of my father William, Will I am, breathing somewhere in my DNA. His life in the theater, that I never knew existed, grew in me like a gorilla in my brain. It is 1972—my day to move into my dorm—and Joy's driving with Bill riding shotgun. Just outside Willard Hall, there's a longhaired hippy, long past college, intoning, "Take a deep breath of air and think about what you have to do next." I think my father inhales that warning into every fingertip: three years later he will expire.

My brother is a year ahead of me at Loyola, on the north side, and we talk on the roof of his apartment building. I'm struggling in Econ and he says easily, Drop the class. This is a concept I cannot begin to comprehend—that would mean failing. He wants to know if I ever just throw things. Like what, I say. A cup and saucer, he says. Anything. I guess I don't. Just throw something, he says. He drives me back on his motorcycle, zigzagging like crazy and I am seriously frightened. He says, If you don't ride it like this, there's no point in riding it at all.

Saturday July 6, 1974 [fourteenth entry]

I can sincerely regret the writings on previous weekends, particularly the ones wherein I stated that my wife + my kids hated me. I am beginning to realize now that when I am having one of these spells, I am an extremely difficult person to live with. Doctor Rovner himself has said on my last few visits that he was more worried about Joy than about me; because during the week, every time the phone rings, Joy is terrified that it might be I, off the deep end again + Joy has to come down + pick me up which is killing her because she has a bad heart + bladder trouble I think I am getting a little better understanding of the psychological aspect of my problem + why they are completely now related to whatever medications I am taking.

And now, incidentally it so happens that the July 4 4 day weekend has really been a bonanza. I was ok all 4 days this holiday weekend. Joy + I went out to lunch one day. I cut the grass front + back yard. We went to Great Lakes one day. We pulled everything down off the back porch, screening beams etc. as that porch is going to be rebuilt with new screening, sideboards etc. Then last night Joy, myself, + Ben + Janice Hinsdale went down to Grant Park for a delightful concert by the Grant Park Symphony Orchestra + George Gershwin. It was a perfect nite, cool, cloudless; I really felt good. The only thing that I must work on is this feeling of independence from Joy. Every time she leaves the house; even when I'm ok I get that uneasy feeling that something might happen to her + that she will not be coming back. I believe that is the crux of the whole situation. I must be able to function on my own—to be my own man. The medication will help but the psychological thing, that evil cancer in my mind, must be destroyed. That is that is that.

WJMcAuliffe

When I see a shrink for the first time at the age of thirty-four in North Carolina, he calls the theme of my life: "violent loss." This sounds accurate, but I'm not sure how it helps me. You're probably wondering why I waited so long. Not only why, but how. What can I say, I should have gone sooner, but Monday morning quarterbacking is always twenty-twenty. We didn't go to shrinks in my house; we talked to priests, or to neurologists who blame problems on lack of willpower. Exorcism might have been an option.

This shrink wisely tells me that my problem with sadness, a black abyss inside me that I am afraid to enter because I don't believe there's any way out of it, is that I have never grieved for my father. I thought it was because I lost my older brother in a motorcycle accident four years after my father died. He asks me to stand in my father's shoes, to see the world from his point of view. He doesn't mean literally stand in his shoes, and anyway, I had already tried that with his magic brown slippers that I wore till they fell apart. I stand in his office and do the dance—spinning like Bill in one of his Saturday spells—the one my little brother and I lapse into whenever we see each other: a kind of secret handshake we only do in private. We dance around in Dad's shoes, or lack thereof because he's usually barefoot in his tracksuit. It's a sick joke between us, a ritual to drive out the demon. When we imitate Bill, we are all together again under the Silly Billy and my father is alive and ill, still good and warm. We conjure him back to life for a few moments and laugh through tears together, back in the insanity of our childhood—the only two left who remember that secret horror film of a world. We can't stand to do it for very long, but we have to do it a little, quote the key phrases: All right then, Jody. Okay then, Jack. You want to fight me, Jody? It's safe to call it hovering—even though my lucid father always insisted, Do not hover!—shifting lightly from one foot to the other, hands out to the side bouncing invisible basketballs, hand to mouth in mild surprise, pat hand to mouth, moan, hand patting door jamb, jamming the walls even though he can't improvise on the clarinet like Benny Goodman. His eyes look terrified. We know how to do the look; we've seen it enough—hell, it's burned onto our retinas. "The angles are all off." That's what he must see, his world tilting. For some reason I cannot fathom, when I do the dance in the shrink's office, when I play my father, I do not feel afraid.

A character created by Don DeLillo—Lauren Hartke (art hidden inside her name) in *The Body Artist*—finds an inevitable and fine-bodied man on the third floor of her rented beach house, a place she's come to grieve alone for her husband, who's committed suicide. Mr. Tuttle, as she names him, carries all the hallmarks of the Boo clan—halting speech, actions of limited ability, shuffling gait, face unfinished, "marked by struggle." He's always in the way, but she can't survive without him—the reflection of death, of the unrealized or under-realized self, the ghost of another reality lurking among us in dream-time, without identity or language, in a state of collapse. He's not a man and not a child, but a channel, existing between the world and the dead, exposing our rawness, aloneness, and fear. He's not crazy, he just can't articulate or comprehend, and in his failure he threatens our assumptions. So, Boo. So, Bill.

Saturday July 13, 1974 [fifteenth entry]

Well, I did it again; this time though it has to be my fault because I don't remember what happened Sunday; all I know is the simple fact though that I must have gone to church; in fact I know though that Joy has confiscated all my medication. And said that she would like to kill myself. [Freudian slip] *Time doesn't permit me to write the whole thing because its Sunday + I have to go to work tomorrow.*

WJMcAuliffe

My shrink says I might accept the love that my mother has to give me, and is there anything about her that I admire. After a brief reflection, I admit that I admire her faith. My shrink draws two overlapping circles. The one is invading the other, the White Tornado–Parnelli Jones Mother is invading the daughter's circle, the mother and the daughter have no sense of boundaries, the daughter can't say no. Rilke says to love is to protect, border, and greet: the shrink draws two circles that touch.

After my father and older brother Brien are dead, my mother says I have no self-esteem, but I have so little that I don't even know what she's talking about. The only thing I'm sure of is that she doesn't know what she's talking about. It's obvious to me now, of course, that she was right about everything. That my boyfriend at that time was a drowned rat and a phony, or a phony who looked like a drowned rat, or just a drowned rat and leave it at that. He's happy to take money from me, but when I send a telegram to him in Poland where he's working, to tell him that my brother is killed, he does not reply. After he returns, he tells me that he didn't reply because he didn't know what to say, and I accept this idiotic explanation because I'm terrified of being alone, so terrified, in fact, that after issuing an ultimatum to him that we get married or break up, I agree to his even more idiotic proposition that we get married without telling anyone, which we, in fact, do. I think I had to marry him to break up with him; I don't know why he suggested this, perhaps hoping I would refuse, but then why did he go through with it? Could it be that he was afraid of losing me, but he still wanted to fool around, or just exhibiting drowned-rat behavior—general, slippery sliminess. I leave for California for work, to get as far away from him as possible without realizing it at the time. We don't live together; he cheats on me; he tells me he wants to be alone; a friend of mine rats him out to me; we get divorced. Through it all, I obstinately cling to the point of view that my mother is wrong about everything. Some things you really do have to learn the hard way.

After some sessions my shrink says I should cry whenever I feel like it and that it's better to cry with other people than alone. I wear my Ray-Bans and cry often, sometimes in groups, mostly singly. I go back to church. There in the pew next to me I see a man of indeterminate age: an ashen, fading, tender, pale, childlike version of my father. Me crying, full of pity for him, and he turns to me beaming, an angel in disguise. I'm the one who needs help, not him.

Saturday 6-15-74 [eleventh entry] *The last week has been one of the most disastrous ones in my history. I am really so confused now that I don't even know what happened. Because it's Saturday again and I am not sure whether I am completely nuts or what in the world is wrong with me whether I should be hospitalized or locked up or what. All I know is that today is today + my job is going to be increasingly difficult Monday if + when I go back to work. It seems to me a century ago that I last went to work. I don't know if I will ever again regain my composure + self reliance again. I hope to God that everything will turn out ok today. I know that Joy hates me + the kids are always against me. I am the one that always is the destroyer. Now the doctor is making out prescriptions for them about me. I don't know I'm so despondent + depressed that I feel like I'd do everybody a favor by dying or committing suicide.*

William McAuliffe

Part Five

The Body—borrows a Revolver—
He bolts the Door—
O'erlooking a superior spectre—
Or More—

C. 1863, EMILY DICKINSON

An Obscure Malady

October 29, 1990, and I'm reading the *New Yorker* and come across an article by Terence Monmaney, "An Epidemic of Brain Disease: This Obscure Malady." I still have the magazine; there's a pumpkin on the cover with a man's face inside of it. Monmaney documents the work of a neuropathologist named Zimmerman—an expert on ALS, known as Lou Gehrig's disease—who was brought to Guam to investigate "diseases of military importance." Torticollis as a disease of military importance? My brother thinks it's only a disease of soldiers.

Zimmerman discovers an inordinately high number of cases of ALS on Guam, where the Japanese notoriously cut off fifty-one heads before the United States takes the island back. Magellan called Guam "the Island of Thieves." The myth about the high incidence on Guam of ALS—called "lytico and bodig"—is that it is the result of a curse. A Catholic priest cursed a native and all his descendants for picking mangos he had been forbidden to harvest: a Catholic conspiracy. In this scenario, disease results from the Catholic attempt to govern the native population of Guam, to bring so-called light into so-called darkness—a plague resulting from an errant empire-building enterprise. In WWII, the navy inadvertently brings tree-climbing snakes hiding in the holds of their ships like stowaways in Trojan horses. The snakes kill and eat all the birds: the island turns silent. The navy destroys music by accident. After the war, doctors find that a large number of Guamanians suffer from a new neurological disorder that acts like a combination of Parkinson's and Alzheimer's—impairing movement and erasing memory. Was it a familial disease? Was it an environmental disease due to diet? My father did not have ALS, but he did have symptoms of both Parkinsonism and dementia. My aunt remembered that his LST routinely stopped in Guam for food supplies.

I write to Monmaney, persuaded, excited, and half hopeful that the secret of my father's mental deterioration lies in the prehistoric jungles of Guam. I clutch at the idea that he may have been poisoned by eating tortillas made from cycad that hadn't been sufficiently detoxified. I know it sounds insane, but there have been cases of "lytico-bodig" after only one taste of cycad and the disease can lie latent like a ticking bomb for decades. I speculate that had he never entered the navy he may never have developed his disease, and if the navy had never landed in Guam, tree-crawling snakes might never have devoured all the birds on the tropical island. They would still be singing. Monmaney writes me back that other children of other WWII soldiers who got their food supplies from Guam have written to him. Their fathers also suffered from neurological disorders.

Recently I discover that the only problem with this theory is that by the time the United States took Guam from the Japanese, Bill had already left the South Pacific. So he couldn't possibly have ingested toxic cycad—a prehistoric plant that looks like part of the set for *Jurassic Park*, a horror movie with dinosaurs, an image of paradise run amuck—the seeds of which kept Guamanians, driven into the jungle by the Japanese, alive. There will be no dinosaurs in my father's horror movie, only humans. Then, four years ago, the *New Yorker* presents the theory of a botanist who posits that it was the eating of a now-extinct bat, a delicacy among native Guamanians, containing an extraordinarily high concentration of cycad, that produced such a high concentration of neurological disease in a population now mostly dead, the secret cause mostly dead with them. The lytico-bodig is vanishing, and my father has vanished before I can decipher him.

Two parts of Monmaney's article still fit my father: brain disease and obscure malady. I reread Oliver Sacks's chapter on Guam in *The Island*. Sacks wonders if the lytico-bodig may have been caused by some sort of virus that came and went: "Some mutant virus, perhaps, with no immediate effect, but affecting people later as their immune systems responded." Sacks describes the sense of community of the native culture on Guam: they treat the afflicted with devotion and compassion. I am reminded of the resentment and irritation I felt at having to respond to my father's repeated questions and irrational behavior. All he heard was shut up, shut up, shut up. I could see the click trip like a circuit breaker as he asked me over and over what day it was, how did he get in the clothes he had on, and clutching the TV guide, asking in mechanical desperation, over and over, why what was written in the TV guide wasn't on the television. This lack of correspondence threatened his grip on reality. I understand now that these repeated questions and verifications were his last-ditch effort to hold onto the present moment. My failure to continuously give the right answer only facilitated the inevitable flip-out that would have to run its course. Yet I know my answering him would not have prevented his dementia. Some unspeakable terror—that I might be looking at my own future—made me want to run.

The Guamanians, on the other hand, accept their sick as people, as part of the community. I loved my father, but he was an embarrassment, a cause of shame, somebody we finally couldn't take care of who needed to be institutionalized. Small wonder he was out on the street in his tracksuit looking for "outside help." I felt overwhelmed at having to make the decision as to where he would go when the VA could no longer keep him. Avoided by us and by the nurses at the VA, he died alone like a rat in a hole, about as far from Tahiti as a person can get.

And what of Tahiti? He used to say that was where he wanted to go. We had a copy of a painting by Gauguin in our house. When I go to the library to find a copy of the painting, at first I can't find it; then several paintings assert themselves, each one trying to persuade me it is the one. Any one could be right and I suddenly fear that I cannot remember, that the image is lost to me: I am losing my balance, becoming confused. Finally there it is—two women with jet-black, luxuriant hair—and I know her immediately, her naked back and half of her left breast before me. The ocean is the skirt she unfolds as a naked girl dives sideways into the waves before her. A headless man spears a fish in the top center. The dream of Tahiti hangs on his living room wall.

Worstward Ho

My friend Alison and I are undergraduates at Northwestern and we decide for some insane—a word I continually abuse: by now you know why—reason to drive to Phoenix and Northern California on U.S. Route 10 in an ancient, yellow Datsun in the dead of summer. That's a ten-year-old yellow Datsun through Death Valley, and her long, thick blonde hair goes all the way down to her butt and I love the way she flips it over her shoulder. By the time we get to Phoenix it's 115 degrees at nine o'clock in the morning and I stand outside at the pool feeling like I'm standing in front of a blast furnace. After nine I can't go outside anymore or I will get skin cancer like my father and his brother. It's in the genes. After dry roasting in Phoenix at her father's, we drive to my brother's in California. We have to stop in the middle of the desert to get out and throw water on the radiator, so overheated that's all we can do to try to cool it down, and as I step out of the car after we pull over, I have the first overpowering sensation that the desert—in all its blasted intensity, clarity, relentlessness, and big sky of endless beauty—is home. The second time I feel that I am spiritually home is in Red Square, the dead of winter, at the height of the Cold War. I'm at home in extremes. We continue up to Santa Cruz on Highway 9—without me knowing that this is the same road on that day in the future when it will be slightly slick from rain, but my big brother will still want to take the Honda motorcycle he has been customizing out for a drive, and on a curve in the road he will slide under a VW bus. They will work on him for two and a half hours, but it won't save him and I wonder if all that working will only make him suffer more. He will not die looking into the eyes of a friend, and the owners of the VW will demand that my mother pay for the damages to their bus, even though they killed my brother. She will pay them because she is honest and fair and bears no grudges. And because she won't know what else to do. There won't be any fight left in her then. What would be the point? Whenever I want to think about my father's death I can't help but think about my brother's death first, even though my father's death happened four years before.

When Alison and I finally find the house in Ben Lomond in the dark, after winding on the 9 and getting lost in the trees, I see a tall shadowy figure leaning in the doorway of a dark wood-frame house hidden in the woods. He looks like Marlon Brando, not fat, just awesome, playing Kurtz in *Apocalypse Now* without bothering or needing to read *Heart of Darkness* or the script, even though that movie hasn't come out yet. My brother wrote psychotic symptoms on his draft form in order to avoid the draft, intuiting from what happened to my father in WWII that Vietnam could cause psychotic symptoms. He turned eighteen on November 17, 1971, and his number was low so it didn't matter that he lied about the symptoms.

I loved my big brother and I told him so in a whisper when I danced with him at his friend David H's wedding. My best friend J slept with him in my parents' bed when they were away and he threw one of his drug parties. I can't imagine where they were because they never went anywhere. I walked into my parents' bedroom looking for J and accidentally saw my brother naked sprawled face up and felt embarrassed. When he died, J's father said to me innocently, He was your first love, wasn't he. Maybe he knows this because his daughter has an older brother, too, and maybe she felt that way about him, or he felt that way about his sister, or maybe he just knows because he can read it in my face.

I think about going out to California to get him and bring him home, but my mother says I should stay at school and keep working. They ship my brother's body cross-country from California to Chicago and my mother is disturbed because the undertaker has combed his hair the wrong way. I fix it so that he looks more like the way he used to look, but his face is strangely bloated. The people he lived with then—he no longer lived in the house in Ben Lomond—send his things to my mother and they feel compelled for some unknown reason to include a dildo in the package. She thinks maybe it's a flashlight so she is spared whatever sick thing it is they are trying to tell her. And some weavings he got in Bolivia. I still have the poncho he got there but I don't wear it anymore. I keep it buried at the bottom of my hopeless chest. I like to know where it is. Woven of horsehair, he's wearing it in the picture with his death crashing toward him like the sea off the coast of Chile, where he looks as if he's on fire. He will be dead in less than a year.

On that day, May 6, 1979, I am in New Haven, a second-year directing student at the Yale School of Drama, in the middle of rehearsals for *The White Devil*, a play about a complicated relationship between a brother and sister. The brother pimps his sister to a duke for money and position. I am in the living room of my apartment perched directly over a bar: at night I need a humidifier to white out the noise. It's the middle of the morning and I am talking to my friend John who's playing Flamineo—"I have a strange thing in me to the which I cannot give a name without it be compassion"—and suddenly I have to lie down because I have a heavy feeling in my chest as if it's being crushed. I tell John I think I am dying, but it's not me who's dying, it's my brother, the one hanging onto the other half of my soul. I lie down on the couch of the apartment I share with the actress playing Vittoria, Flamineo's sister, in the middle of the morning and sleep the sleep of the dead, but only for a few hours. The ringing phone drags me up from under and it's my younger brother telling me that my older brother has been in an accident: He didn't make it. I ask if he was high and he wants to know what difference it makes. He's right, of course. It makes no difference.

The Beginning of the End

> It seems that the honor of a family requires the disappearance from society of the individual who by vile and abject habits shames his relatives.
>
> *Madness and Civilization*, FOUCAULT

My mother has a hysterectomy in 1975, and my older brother has escaped, but not for long, to school in California—that leaves me, twenty years old, in charge. She tells me they can no longer keep Bill at the VA: he will have to go to Downey. She sends me to the VA to take care of the arrangements. He's finally, officially, a leper. Running out in the street in his tracksuit one too many times is probably what did it, but that's really only the tip of the iceberg and we are all on the *Titanic* jockeying for a position in the tiny lifeboat. All the doors and windows in Bill's brain are flapping open and we can't shut them any more. I'm convinced he has to be confined, but I don't even know the dreaded Downey is actually another VA hospital that takes vets for long-term psychiatric care. I know we're talking about warehousing because I grew up on all those movies that scared the shit out of me, along with my mother's tales from the locked ward. I think Downey is a state mental institution even though my father's decline coincides with the end of institutionalization as it has been known. My wry father, lover of the plays of Tennessee Williams, would have appreciated the irony of my reluctant Stella Kowalski to his even more reluctant Blanche Dubois, Williams's monumental, tragic characters in *A Streetcar Named Desire.*

> Stella: What have I done to my sister? Oh, God, what have I done to my sister?
> Eunice: You done the right thing, the only thing you could do. She couldn't stay here; there wasn't no other place for her to go.

At the end of the play, strangers, on whose kindness Blanche has come to depend, lead her off to the nuthouse, "as if she were blind." Here at the VA the strangers are not particularly kind and neither is the daughter. I have not been kind.

My father knows well what his life is like at the VA—he can easily deduce from that experience what it will be like at the closed world of Downey, in the real looney bin, not the cushy looney bin off Michigan Avenue where I can take him on day passes for chocolate sodas. He was forever being moved—from Mercy Hospital in Chicago to the VA when I was born, from Passavant to the VA, and from one VA hospital to Downey if he doesn't die first, which is what he does—and always ending up back with the navy obligated to take him, the navy where the inevitable decline started in the first place, inside the closed world of the ship. They broke him. They're paying for him.

[Wo]Man under the Influence

In 1974, my mother and I see Cassavetes's *A Woman under the Influence.* In this story of a nervous breakdown, a working-class housewife and mother falls apart, gets committed, and comes home to her family, a shadow of her former self. The experience is so intense that I feel as if I must run from the theater. Except I can't move. That's my life up there, my father as Gena Rowlands. It starts with men up to their waists in water, gesturing compulsively, smoking, listening to opera. Then there's Gena, delicate, sensitive, unusual—code for nuts. Husband Peter Falk insists Mabel's not crazy because the woman cooks, sews, washes the bathroom. But she's nervous, insecure—wacko. Puts her fists up: You want to fight me, Jody? Falk says be yourself and she wants him to stand up for her. I did not stand up for my Dad. She dances on the couch to Swan Lake. Dad loves ballet, too. Falk slaps her in front of the kids, knocking her off the sofa. Mom employs the kick-punch method. Mabel says, I'm a grown-up. The chaos level, the violence, the interference from extended family—Cassavetes's actual mother plays Mabel's mother-in-law pushing for commitment—it plays like a documentary of my life, a horror film.

When I get to the VA hospital in the summer of '75, a female social worker corners me as the only viable responsible party and tells me my father has been complaining that my mother won't have sex with him, as if that's the whole problem in a nutshell. Is Bill just telling this woman what she wants to hear, a standard excuse, or has he actually convinced himself that this is the cause? She has got to be kidding. This beyond-ridiculous scene feels straight out of Milos Forman's film of Ken Kesey's novel, *One Flew Over the Cuckoo's Nest.* The film doesn't even come out until three months after my father is dead, November of 1975, but I might as well be in it. Or is this a real factor that I cannot grasp because I don't want to think about my parents' sexual relationship or lack thereof? McMurphy the rebel, in order to get out of jail, fakes his way into a mental institution, only to come up against a formidable nemesis, Big Nurse Ratched. Big Nurse runs the locked ward, brooking no opposition. She wants to talk about Mr. Harding's problem in group therapy: his wife and her big tits making him feel inferior. My father, like Harding—intellectual, sensitive, intimidated by his big-titted wife's sexuality. Harding, when you get right down to it, actually prefers life inside the institution, inside the chain-link fence. It's safer. Bill is no McMurphy, even though McMurphy just wants to play with the word "touching" as in touching on the subject, as in touching Harding's wife's big tits. Bill likes to play with words. And from what I gather from my mother, he must have liked to play with tits—or bazooms as he liked to call them—even though he professed to be a legman. My current dementia research tells me that hypersexuality could be a symptom of Bill's neurological disease.

Fast forward to the winter of 1977: I'm a student in Moscow attending a private screening of *Cuckoo's Nest* at Dom Kino for professionals in the film business. The film is not shown publicly here, it's too close to the bone, too explosive. The atmosphere in the room is electrifying, like a little bit of communal brain burn—political shock treatment for the intelligentsia. Everybody in there, including me, thinks the film is about his life. I even look at wild-eyed Jack Nicholson with prejudice: he seems to have a little bit of a problem with violence. Hijacked into oblivion—but not without guilt.

So the gorilla with the gun is taking over the last room in my father's brain. Downey is not a tolerable option as far as he is concerned. Through a glass partition, the thin membrane between the psychiatric patients and those of us so-called sane, I see my father hovering in the background, waiting as the social worker discusses his case with me. As I fumble through decisions about his fate, I see his haunted eyes shining beyond the glass—backed into a corner. I know this woman has no idea what she's dealing with because your wife not sleeping with you cannot cause catatonia, aphasia, psychotic symptoms, brain damage, or dementia. My language deserts me. I realize I cannot save him.

I explain to this social worker that my mother has just had a hysterectomy, but I am so out of my element—I don't want to be thinking about, let alone discussing, my parents' sex life, whatever is left of it. Once my mother told me I was an accident and that my younger brother was planned. I reorganized these facts in my personal narrative, convincing myself of the opposite: I become planned and he's an accident. Years later I get confused and ask her which is which. She says I was conceived one night because my father wouldn't take no for an answer. According to her, he could be quite determined. Because she was nursing my older brother, she was supposed to not be fertile. My brother and I were almost Irish twins, born within the same year, missed it by a week, but I like the idea that I was conceived out of my father's determination. She laughed, confiding that I once walked in on them in the midst of the act of love. I had no idea.

My father still hovers in the background, behind the glass partition, his look now terrified, like his eyes have relocated to different parts of his head and I know we aren't seeing things the same way. He knows what I'm doing there, and I have to hand it to him: this is an inspired last-ditch attempt to avoid the inevitable. Blame it on Joy. What happened to that laudatory stuff about not siphoning off responsibility onto his wife?

Dear Mom,

I had been getting the impression from your letters that Bill was getting better. From your last letter tho I can understand that he is worse and continuing to worsen. I don't know what the Doctor is saying about it but when he starts wetting the floor it is really out of hand.

It is really impossible to live with someone who can't deal with reality, and I for one do not expect you to, nor do I approve of your doing it as it is going to loosen your own grip. Obviously a solution has to be reached so that you can live without having to be a 24-hour psychiatric nurse. I know he needs help + care and attention but you can't think you are the one who must always provide it.

I'm sure Jack does want to leave but he has to take care of himself too. I wouldn't sell your house, it is beautiful and selling it would not solve the problem. Jody has told me that she really thinks there is far too much strain on you lately. In order to take care of yourself, if you must get away from Bill then do it. It's the same old story about someone swimming out to a drowning victim and then drowning himself. 2 is worse than 1. I don't see what you can do for him, because if you haven't been able to do it by now, I don't know.

He must have needed a place to hide, he used to say he'd be dead by 50. Well he didn't die but he did turn himself off. He must have his reasons, even if he can't say what they are.

Take it more easily

Love Brien [my older brother, deceased]

I find this letter among my mother's papers after her death. I have no memory of Bill wetting the floor so this must have occurred while I was away at college and my mother did not tell me. I am not sure what Brien means by Bill having needed a place to hide. Hide from what exactly? Himself? The world? My mother? All of the above? The main dilemma in the quest for understanding what was wrong with my father is the question of how to or whether to separate organic from psychological symptoms. James L. Halliday of Scotland, writing in 1937 on "Psychological Factors in Rheumatism," seems ahead of his time in his understanding of the necessity to encounter disease as an experience in the body, but also in the mind in the form of fearful knowledge. Dr. Halliday discusses four major questions involved in diagnosis: 1) What kind of person was he? 2) Why did he fall ill when he did? 3) Why did he fall ill in the way he did? 4) Had he any purpose in being ill?

Brien means Bill's purpose in being ill was to hide inside the madness or dementia itself. My brother, like all of us, believed, however wrongly, that my father of his own volition turned himself off—pulled the switch and cut the power. An act of will. Because we thought we could see it happen. Like watching an eclipse and just as damaging and painful to look at. Brien assumes that my father has reasons—this assumes he's rational—even if he can't say what they are. He definitely can't; sometimes he can't even talk—it's called aphasia.

Saturday July 22, 1974 [sixteenth and penultimate entry]

Well, this is another ripoff of a weekend. I still don't know whether it happens Saturday or Sunday but I do know that there was a lot of violence + that it was all my fault. I can't remember everything, but I know that I went off the deep end either Saturday or Sunday + had Jack + Jody sorry that they ever lived here. Then, I guess Brien was disgusted with my performance the other weekend. If I could only sort it all out I know that with the medication properly taken I should be able to keep myself under control. I'll try my damnest now to keep myself under control.

WJMcAuliffe

Dad, in one of your lucid moments—you did still have them—in March 1975, six months before you will expire, I sit with you as you are lying down on Mom's half of your narrow double bed in this, the last room that still belongs to you, and you tell me what you know at fifty-four: that there is nothing left for you to do but die. I hold your right hand just as I held Mom's left hand in August of 2005 as she died saying, Let me go. But I am not there for the real thing for you: You do not tell me you're glad I'm here at your bedside in the psycho ward at the VA and I'm not holding your hand. I was not there. It's the middle of the night and I'm driving up winding coastal highway 9, my brother's future graveyard, or I'm seeing the Pacific for the first time through the fog at dawn. You die alone.

Dementia

Dementia is Pinel's term. He arranged mental diseases into three categories: 1) Mania, 2) Melancholia, 3) Demency, or a particular debility of the operations of the understanding, and of the acts of the will. If you're demented, you've had your mind removed and maybe your will, too. Willis, the seventeenth-century physician and brain anatomist, recognized the kinship between melancholy and madness: these distempers often change and pass from one into the other. Depression leads to agitation; agitation to depression. Torticollis, a spasm, would have fallen under Willis's hysterical symptoms. Willis knew men without wombs had so-called hysterical symptoms, and women with healthy wombs had so-called hysterical symptoms. Though he recognized the role of emotion in the cause of illness, he concluded that hysterical symptoms arose in the brain, from disturbance in "hinder parts" at the beginnings of the nerves in the head. Willis was well on his way to holding the basal ganglia responsible for torticollis.

By 1971, four years before my father's death, no one doubts that the disease of torticollis is NOT psychogenic in origin. Today, investigators believe that the dystonias, including torticollis, result from an abnormality in an area of the brain called the basal ganglia, where some of the messages that initiate muscle contractions are processed. Scientists suspect a defect in the body's ability to process a group of chemicals, called neurotransmitters, that help cells in the brain communicate with each other, but the cause remains unknown.

Pinel says, "It has been already observed, that people of great warmth of imagination, acuteness of sensibility and violence of passions, are most predisposed to insanity." In Bill's case, Pinel would have recognized the traumatic and neurological causes along with the stress factor. I wonder if half of my father's problem stemmed from the stress of living at home with us, and the other half was neurological. If only he had stayed in the theater, he could have lived in imaginary worlds. Fine arts help manage the insane.

Still no autopsy: What's wrong with his brain? Good luck.

Pinel: *I have no where met, excepting in romances, with fonder husbands, more affectionate parents, more impassioned lovers, more pure and exalted patriots, than in the lunatic asylum, during their intervals of calmness and reason. A man of sensibility may go there every day of his life, and witness scenes of indescribable tenderness associated to a most estimable virtue.*

An old friend of mine has a brother who's a neurologist. His best estimate is that my father had something called Lewy body disease. The giveaways are his pronounced hallucinations, fluctuations in cognitive status, and the "bad" response to antipsychotics—Thorazine, Mellaril, and Haldol, the three that I can remember him taking; and don't forget the tremor—significantly without slow movement and muscle rigidity. Antipsychotics sent Bill into severe mental tailspins. Apparently, Lewy body patients have a paradoxical response to phenothiazines. These drugs make them much worse. I have long wondered whether Bill had Parkinsonian dementia, even though his only Parkinsonian symptom was the tremor. The neurologist tells me that Parkinsonian dementia sets in when the body freezes, and the only thing freezing on my father was his mind. Half dead at the top.

Dad,

I really think you ought to consider the implications of the Thorazine. It obviously does not help, I would advise you not to take it. I really can't see how these tranquilizers are doing you any good. They seem to confuse and agitate you even more. I really think you ought to follow up on the yoga relaxing exercises and try to learn to control your body more. Drugs will obviously not work in your case (tranquilizers that is, not artane [for parkinsonism]*). The doctor ought to be confronted with this reaction that you have, tell him what happens to you. You are going to have to work harder on yourself and stop depending on the drugs to keep your feet on the ground.*

Let a little peace into yourself where & whenever you find room or a chance.
Love, Brien

Take responsibility for your madness.

I agree that his history doesn't suggest Parkinson's. His spells lasted sometimes a day or part of a day, sometimes the whole weekend; they got longer and longer and I think that sleep was required for him to maybe get back to something like normal the next day, with no memory of the day before except that he knew he had "flipped out." Lewy body patients can have lucid moments. The fact that he couldn't dress himself was also a symptom. And here I thought he just didn't like what my mother picked out for him. She liked maroon and velour and he did not. He looks down at himself and pulls at his clothes, "I just need to get out of these offensive clothes."

In the final year he corners me in the hall outside the bathroom. It's hard for me to believe today that the five of us lived in a house with only one bathroom. It's a wonder we didn't all kill each other. One time he tries to get in the bathroom while Brien is in there on the toilet. Bill pushes the unlockable door in on him and Brien slams it so hard he almost takes my father's finger off in the hinge. It's hanging by a thread. This is one of his infamous visits to the emergency room that's actually necessary. When you suffer from anxiety and hypochondria, you endure many false ER alarms. This time, Bill doesn't have to be embarrassed once he arrives cradling his wounded flesh, not like the time the chest pains evaporate into thin air and he feels like a fool.

He corners me outside the one bathroom. It's no accident that this is the scene of some heavy confrontations. At this point I outweigh him: he's 5'10" and down to 125 pounds. He says, You want to fight me, Jody? and puts up his dukes. Remember, he boxed in high school. I have trouble imagining it but it's right there in the yearbook, on the team no less, but now his postsurgical shoulders are frozen in a U-shaped curve like a yoke. In the old presurgery post-torticollis pictures he's got these big broad shoulders and big grin—now that guy could box!—it's hard to believe this is the same person. He's so light on his feet I feel like I could blow on him and he'd fall over. I don't know whether to laugh or cry. Now I find out heightened belligerence is a symptom of dementia, but I don't know that at the time. All I know is I don't want to fight him. I'd like to kill him because he's driving me nuts, but I don't want to hurt him.

The term "Lewy body" rings an ominous bell in my head, maybe from my obsessive research on mad-cow disease. More armchair neurology. More heightened fears of inexplicable brain deterioration, more fears of the hidden heredity time bomb. My neurologist friend disagrees with Dr. Rovner's diagnosis of willpower and anxiety, and thinks that Bill was likely suffering from dementia at that time. I don't know if I'm scared or relieved, but I have to believe it. He does not, regrettably, humor me in my fantasy that there is some deep connection between torticollis + surgery + tremor + cognitive decline = dementia, but I refuse to surrender the aesthetic comfort of this dramatic progression. Torticollis could have pathologized his personality, turning spasmodic torticollis into mental torticollis, a disease of anxiety, guilt, or both. The mind has a beautiful way of adapting. The neurologist does have an explanation for why the Saturday breakdowns: the structure of the workweek and workplace oriented my father, while the weekend brought out his dementia. His confusionary spells began on Saturdays when he wasn't working. But then the spells started happening when he was at work. The dementia was taking over.

When I tell my friend that my father was forty-five when the confusion started and fifty-four when he died, he observes that that's young for Lewy body disease. He warns that in someone that young, the differential broadens considerably and includes neurogenetic disease. Sounds ominous. Remind me not to get tested. Since 1975 preceded the MRI, he wonders if Bill ever got a spinal tap to exclude an inflammatory/infectious etiology, and wants to know the ultimate cause of death. I don't remember any spinal tap and I'm sure I would have heard about it because that would have been quite painful. My father's pain threshold, like mine—we're both redheads—is exceptionally low. Our collective skin is thin and the capillaries close to the surface, even though the feelings are submerged twenty thousand leagues under the sea.

Now, as a writer trying to understand, I feel as if I am back to square one. I thought Lewy body disease was the answer I am looking for, even if it's only a scientific name that refuses the comfort of catharsis. The name can't erase the suffering, any more than the gas-chamber execution of Pixley can bring my cousins back to life.

I get *Early-Onset Dementia* from the library and discover that urinary incontinence is a symptom of dementia with Lewy bodies. Along with rapid cognitive decline. Lewy body disease has been reported to occur before the age of fifty. Death occurs five years from onset.

I decide that I believe he had Lewy body dementia. I know it wasn't his fault. He was a good father, my best and only.

July 14, 1975

Dear Dad,
I've talked to Mom on the phone and she said the doctors had taken you off all medication and that you were in an oxygen tent on intravenous. I hope you are doing better now and are able to eat and drink yourself. However difficult it may seem they are doing something that should have been done long ago.

I just want you to know that I am with you spiritually and that I hope that means something to you. You have a long way to go, I hope you can and want to, keep on with it.

At least you are still closeby, and Grandma & Mary can see you as well as Mom & kids. I will be home in September sometime, so I will see you then.

At any rate I hope you feel like you've got a better hold on things in your life than you have before.

I have not heard from you in a while, and I don't know if you are still writing letters. But I would like to hear from you how you are instead of having everybody else's opinions and comments.
Love Brien

Six weeks later my father was dead.

10-18-73

Dear Jody,
As you can immediately ascertain, this stationery I'm using is of a rather curious nature. These are our job order forms + the ones I'm using are out of date. So in between interviewing alcoholics this afternoon (it's kind of a slow day) I thought I would drop a few lines to my daughter to see how she is coming along.

My recent vacation was anything but a complete bust. Joy + I went out once with grandma to Stouffers; then on the last Sunday before I went back to work Joy + I went to dinner at The Flame; + in between dining on the town we made a very interesting trip to the Museum of Science + Industry, where I made my fourth trip through the U505 German submarine, saw Coleen Moore's famous doll's house, saw the Ringling Bros. Barnum + Bailey circus in miniature + a brief but stunning movie on circus life.

Your last letter was enjoyed by all of us, + I was glad to hear that you're doing so well in gymnastics + speech.

Don't worry too much about your feelings of insecurity. You know that we all love you; that you have a bevy of good friends. One thing that I do know, though, is that the experience of living from day to day, will never, + can never quite measure up to what we expect out of life. On the other hand, feelings that we at first had extraordinary difficulty in expressing or repressing often bloom into experiences of amazing beauty + richness.

On looking at yourself with complete honesty, Jo, you know that you have rare talents, physical + mental, going for you. Make the best of these + you will find that your neuroses will take care of themselves. The whole world is slightly neurotic these days.

Love,
Dad

Once, I thought of abandoning my vocation and going to law school. I stopped into a church in Santa Monica and sat in a pew in the dark next to a pillar. After awhile, I feel my father on one side of me and my brother on the other. They say I shouldn't let other people drive me away from what I want to do. I know they're dead but I believe in ghosts. My husband says the way I am with them makes them live forever.

I still miss my father. I missed him while he was alive. These days when I talk to my brother on the phone, I can say the words, and conjure him: OK, then, too; alright, then; today IS Saturday; I am having difficulty in articulation; all I want is some reassurance, as you well know . . . a place for everything and everything in its place; just checking; I need outside help; the angles are all off; no phone calls during the dinner hour; your mother has destroyed the evidence of dinner . . . the disintegration of the family unit . . . I was an officer in the Japanese navy, and was shot in the back of the neck while trying to escape; the higher the fewer; I was an officer in the German air force, and was shot in the back of the neck while trying to escape; I believe there is a plot afoot; I value my family more than my own life; well so much for now though.

I still have some of his stuff: his military ID bracelet, his navy pins, his Notre Dame bracelet, his high school pendant, evening scarves and silk handkerchiefs; his penny box, falling apart at the hinges, held together with a thick rubber band, where we got silver dollars to buy Good Humor bars from the man in the truck; the china dog with his nose and tail in the air that he hung his watch on, his Hamilton mechanical watch, repaired until it could no longer be fixed. I don't know where it is or what I did with it. I bought one that resembled it, but it's just not the same. I want the old one back. I want to hold it to my ear and hear it tick.

Acknowledgments

I am grateful for reactions to the manuscript given to me by Allan Havis, W. D. King, Jeff Jackson, Corina Stan, Tom DiPietro, Don DeLillo, Elizabeth Davis, Marlane Meyer, Victoria Christian, and Frank Lentricchia. I wish to thank Dr. Lawrence Greenblatt, Dr. Peter King, neurologist, and Candy Conino, physical therapist and Feldenkrais practitioner, for their invaluable assistance; William Noland, for preparing the photographs for publication; and Joe Parsons, formerly at the University of Iowa Press and now at the University of North Carolina Press, for his recognition of and enthusiasm for my work.

An early version of Part One appeared in *Topograph: New Writing from the Carolinas and the Landscape Beyond*, edited by Jeff Jackson (Novello Festival Press, 2010). A few fragments from my short story, *Standing on End*, originally published in *Southwest Review*, make an appearance in parts three and four.

Appendix

A Brief History of Surgical Approaches to Torticollis

Second century A.D.: Antyllus, a Greek surgeon, practices tenotomy, the cutting or dividing of a tendon.

Medieval era: Itinerant practitioners—charlatans, quacks, and mountebanks— perform tenotomy, cymbals clanging to drown out cries of patients.

Fabricius of Padua (1537–1619): Anatomist, surgeon, and tutor of William Harvey (who first described circulation of the blood), he devises a brace for correction of the deformity.

1641: Isaac Minnius, a German army surgeon, attempts surgical correction, the first reported open section of the sternomastoid muscle for the relief of the affection, torticollis. Note: "Affection" is used here by Finney and Hughson in 1925. Affection, from the Latin *affectio*, a state of feeling: a mental or emotional state or tendency; [Archaic] a disease; ailment—SYNONYM LOVE.

1641: Nicolaas Tulp gives anatomy lessons, performing them on victims of public hanging; wry-neck day is hanging day. Rembrandt paints *Anatomy Lesson of Nicolaas Tulp*, in which only one of the council and guild members required to attend, and to pay for the privilege, actually looks at Dr. Tulp's dissection of the executed criminal's forearm. Tulp looks like a priest. He writes about muscular wry-neck in *The Book of Monsters* (1641).

1648–79: John Ward, in his diary for this time period, writes of a quack who divides "three tendons in a child's neck, making a small incision with a lancet and elevating the tendon for fear of wounding the jugular vein and inserting a knife to divide the tendon 'upwards' with a loud snap." (David LeVay, *The History of Orthopaedics*)

1652: Physician Tulp consults surgeon Minnius about his operation on a 12-year-old boy for congenital torticollis and describes the surgery in his *Observationes*. Minnius, the first to do this operation, divides "the muscle over the clavicle with a knife 'from the ear towards the throat'." J. F. Dieffenbach, author of "On the Cure of Wry Neck," remarks that Minnius secures "immortality merely by thinking of this unconventional procedure," and adds that "by placing a skin scar over the muscle," Minnius does "everything likely to bring about a recurrence." (LeVay)

Job van Meek'ren (1611–66): Describes Florianus' operation "on a 14-year-old boy, tied to a chair and held down" while the tendon "gave such a snap . . . as if one had plucked the string of a musical instrument." (LeVay)

1670: Obstetrician Hendrick Van Roonhuysen, who invented a secret lever for delivering a baby stuck during birth, performs several operations for wry-neck and describes surgical correction: "It was our great good fortune that our little knife was rather broad and blunt at the back, for otherwise we might easily have damaged the windpipe and the artery, which were most plainly to be seen the following day, from which it may be sufficiently deduced how dangerous and destructive it would be to use caustic or corrosive agents . . . and how cautiously the knife must be used and everything kept ready for a severe haemorrhage, which could so easily follow." (LeVay)

1696: Antonius Nuck uses a "head suspension appliance called the torques," though he admits that surgery has its place. (LeVay)

1737: Von Jaeger's inaugural dissertation at Tubingen is titled *Torticollis.*

1768: Samuel Sharpe uses a button-ended knife to divide the sternomastoid tendon from within outwards: "After the Incision is made, the wound is to be . . . dressed so as to prevent the extremities of the Muscle from reuniting; to which end they are to be separated from each other as much as possible by the assistance of a supporting Bandage for the Head during the whole time of the Cure, which will generally be about a Month." (Sharpe, *A Treatise on the Operations of Surgery*)

1810: Johann C. F. Jorg believes that operative treatment of torticollis "might have been suitable for a cruder age, but that every case could be cured by his own ingenious device in which a head-band was connected to a breastplate by a ratchet." (LeVay)

1812: Baron Guillaume Dupuytren, a famous military surgeon, performs first closed tenotomy of the sternocleidomastoid muscle at its sternal origin. The shoulder is "brought down by tying the right hand to the right foot." (LeVay) Several fatalities from damage to underlying vessels ensue. Open operation becomes method of choice.

1825: No surgeon yet knows the cause(s) of spasmodic torticollis.

1834: Bujalski resects, removes part of, both spinal accessory nerves in a case of bilateral spasm of the sternomastoids. Nobody takes note.

1866: Campbell de Morgan of London advances by attacking nerve supply to the muscles—performing section of the spinal accessory nerve. Some favor nerve stretching or constriction of the nerve trunk with silver wire, with success stories recorded. Note: American and English physicians prefer surgical attack via nerve route; Germans choose muscle route.

1891: W. W. Keen cuts the muscles, but only in order to divide the motor nerve supply. Finney and Hughson consider this the first "carefully studied and scientific attempt to treat the disease on a rational basis."

1912: Kocher pushes multiple myotomy—division of sternomastoid and transverse incision across the back of the neck to divide the muscles that rotate the head. He and his partner believe that dividing the muscles, to interfere with the cortical stimuli, will prevent the muscle "habit"—a pattern of action that is acquired and has become so automatic that it is difficult to break—from returning.

1925: John Finney and Walter Hughson, who stress the neurotic or psychopathic factor in some cases, develop Keen's idea: excise the nerve supply of all "offending" muscles to guarantee the end of spasm in them.

1925: No surgeon yet knows the cause(s) of spasmodic torticollis.

1930: W. E. Dandy first describes "bilateral intraspinal division of the roots of the first three cervical roots and the intracranial division of the spinal accessory nerve, with excellent results in five out of eight patients." (Mark A. Stacy, *Handbook of Dystonia*)

1955: K. G. McKenzie "advocates peripheral sectioning of the accessory nerve to the sternocleidomastoid be added to the intraspinal procedure." Dandy-McKenzie remains "procedure of choice until the late 1970s." (Stacy)

1978: C. Bertrand develops "a more benign treatment," identifying "the muscles to be denervated for the different types of torticollis." (Stacy)

1986: H. J. Colbassani Jr. and J. H. Wood "warn of significant risks" to Dandy-McKenzie procedure. (Stacy)

2010: Surgery is rarely used to treat spasmodic torticollis, no longer thought to be a psychiatric disorder, but rather caused by a dysfunction in the part of the brain that handles muscle contraction messages. Surgery to remove muscle motor nerves involved in contraction and deep brain stimulation—a pacemaker for the brain—are options of last resort. There is no cure.

A Short Bibliography of Works Consulted and Cited

Aamodt, Sandra, and Sam Wang. *Welcome to Your Brain.* New York: Bloomsbury, 2008.

Baldwin, James. *The Fire Next Time.* New York: Dial Press, 1963.

Bergson, Henri. *Laughter: An Essay on the Meaning of the Comic.* New York: Macmillan, 1928.

Brecht, Bertolt. *Collected Plays.* New York: Vintage Books, 1971.

Cheyne, George. *A Treatise of Nervous Diseases of All Kinds.* London: Printed for G. Strahan in Cornhill, 1733.

Clark, L. P. "The Results of the Psychic Treatment of Mental Torticollis." *Medical Record* 92 (July 14, 1917): 48–54.

DeLillo, Don. *The Body Artist.* New York: Scribner, 2001.

Dickinson, Emily. *Poems of Emily Dickinson.* Edited by T. W. Higginson and Mabel Loomis Todd. Boston: Little, Brown, 1910.

Durrenmatt, Friedrich. *The Physicists.* New York: Grove Press, 1964.

Finney, John, and Walter Hughson. "Spasmodic Torticollis." *Annals of Surgery* 81 (January 1925): 255–69.

Foucault, Michel. *Madness and Civilization: A History of Insanity in the Age of Reason.* New York: Random House, 1965.

"Girls' Slaying Suspect Gives Insanity Plea." *Chicago Tribune.* September 24, 1964.

Goffman, Erving. *Asylums: Essays on the Social Situation of Mental Patients and Other Inmates.* New York: Anchor Books, 1961.

———. *Stigma: Notes on the Management of Spoiled Identity.* New Jersey: Prentice-Hall, 1963.

Gowers, W. R. *A Manual of Diseases of the Nervous System.* Philadelphia: Blakiston, 1897–98.

Griffin, John Howard. *Black Like Me.* New York: New American Library, 1960.

Grinker, Roy R., and John P. Spiegel. *Men under Stress*. Philadelphia: Blakiston, 1945.

Halliday, James L. "Psychological Factors in Rheumatism, Part 1." *British Medical Journal* 1 (February 6, 1937): 264–69.

Hemingway, Ernest. *The Short Stories of Ernest Hemingway*. New York: Scribner, 1925.

Hodges, John R., ed. *Early-Onset Dementia: A Multidisciplinary Approach*. Oxford: Oxford University Press, 2001.

"Hysterical Wry Neck of Soldiers." *Journal of the Association of Military Surgeons of the United States* 97 (1945): 59–60.

Ibsen, Henrik. *John Gabriel Borkman*. London: Nick Hern, 1997.

In re Robert E. McAuliffe, Attorney, Respondent, No. 63424, Supreme Court of Illinois, 116 Ill. 2d 254; 506 N.E.2d 1300; 1987 Ill. LEXIS 175; 107 Ill. Dec. 245, February 20, 1987, Filed.

Journal of Neurological Science 4 (1967): 1–13.

"Judge Nabs Killer of Daughters." *Chicago Tribune*. August 8, 1964.

"Judge, Wife, Last Child on Sad Trip Home." *Chicago Tribune*. August 9, 1964.

Kafka, Franz. *The Metamorphosis and Other Stories*. New York: Oxford University Press, 2009.

Latham, R. G. *The Works of Thomas Sydenham, MD*. London: C. and J. Adlard, 1750.

Lee, Harper. *To Kill a Mockingbird*. New York: Harper Collins, 1999.

Lees, A. J. *Tics and Related Disorders*. Edinburgh: Elsevier Health Sciences, 1986.

Lentricchia, Frank, and Jody McAuliffe. *Crimes of Art + Terror*. Chicago: University of Chicago Press, 2003.

LeVay, David. *The History of Orthopaedics: An Account of the Study and Practice of Orthopaedics from the Earliest Times to the Modern Era*. Park Ridge, NJ: Parthenon, 1990.

Mandel, Oscar. *Philoctetes and the Fall of Troy*. Lincoln: University of Nebraska Press, 1981.

Matz, Terry. *The Daybook of the Saints*. New York: Viking, 2001.

McAuliffe, Jody. "Standing on End." *Southwest Review* (Spring 1989): 262–66.

Merskey, Harold. *The Analysis of Hysteria: Understanding Conversion and Dissociation*. London: Gaskell, 1995.

Monmaney, Terence. "An Epidemic of Brain Disease: This Obscure Malady." *New Yorker* (October 29, 1990): 85–101.

O'Brien, John, David Ames, and Alistair Burns, eds. *Dementia.* New York: Oxford University Press, 2000.

Pinel, Philippe. *Treatise on Insanity.* Washington, DC: University Publications of America, 1977.

Plutarch. *Greek Lives.* Oxford: Oxford University Press, 2009.

Rabelais, Francois. *Gargantua and Pantagruel.* New York: Norton, 1990.

Risher, Arthur L. "Torticollis: A Review." *Journal of Bone and Joint Surgery* (1916): 669–81.

Russell, Ray. *Sardonicus and Other Stories.* New York: Ballantine, 1961.

Sacks, Oliver. *The Island of the Colorblind.* New York: Knopf, 1996.

Scaer, Robert. *The Body Bears the Burden: Trauma, Dissociation, and Disease.* Rochester, MN: Haworth Press, 2007.

"Services Held for Judge's Two Daughters." *Chicago Tribune.* August 14, 1964.

Sherrod, Robert. *Tarawa: The Story of a Battle.* New York: Duell, Sloan and Pearce, 1944.

"Slain Girls' Kin Returns from Wyoming." *Chicago Tribune.* August 10, 1964.

Sontag, Susan. *Illness as Metaphor.* New York: Farrar, Straus and Giroux, 2001.

Spillane, John David. *The Doctrine of the Nerves: Chapters in the History of Neurology.* Oxford: Oxford University Press, 1981.

Stacy, Mark A., ed. *Handbook of Dystonia.* New York: Informa Healthcare, 2007.

"Suspect Given 'Truth Serum' in Death Quiz." *Chicago Tribune.* August 11, 1964.

Whiles, W. H. "Treatment of Spasmodic Torticollis by Psychotherapy." *British Medical Journal* (June 15, 1940): 969–71.

Whisler, Weldon. "Sad Parents of Slain Girls Tell of Faith." *Chicago Tribune.* August 3, 1964.

Wiener, Jonathan. "The Tangle: Searching for the Cause of a Brain Disease." *New Yorker* (April 11, 2005): 42–51.

Willis, Thomas. *The Anatomy of the Brain and Nerves.* Birmingham, AL: Classics of Neurology & Neurosurgery Library, 1983.

sightline books

The Iowa Series in Literary Nonfiction

The Men in My Country
MARILYN ABILDSKOV

Shadow Girl: A Memoir of Attachment
DEB ABRAMSON

Anthropologies: A Family Memoir
BETH ALVARADO

On the Shoreline of Knowledge: Irish Wanderings
CHRIS ARTHUR

Embalming Mom: Essays in Life
JANET BURROWAY

Family Bible
MELISSA J. DELBRIDGE

Dream Not of Other Worlds: Teaching in a Segregated Elementary School, 1970
HUSTON DIEHL

Fauna and Flora, Earth and Sky: Brushes with Nature's Wisdom
TRUDY DITTMAR

Little Big World: Collecting Louis Marx and the American Fifties
JEFFREY HAMMOND

In Defense of Nature
JOHN HAY

Stories We Tell Ourselves: "Dream Life" and "Seeing Things"
MICHELLE HERMAN

Trespasses: A Memoir
LACY M. JOHNSON

Letters to Kate: Life after Life
CARL H. KLAUS

Desert Year
JOSEPH WOOD KRUTCH

The Great Chain of Life
JOSEPH WOOD KRUTCH

Essays of Elia
CHARLES LAMB

The Body of Brooklyn
DAVID LAZAR

In Earshot of Water: Notes from the Columbia Plateau
PAUL LINDHOLDT

No Such Country: Essays toward Home
ELMAR LUETH

The Mythical Bill: A Neurological Memoir
JODY MCAULIFFE

Grammar Lessons: Translating a Life in Spain
MICHELE MORANO

Currency of the Heart: A Year of Investing, Death, Work, and Coins
DONALD R. NICHOLS

In the Memory of the Map: A Cartographic Memoir
CHRISTOPHER NORMENT

Return to Warden's Grove: Science, Desire, and the Lives of Sparrows
CHRISTOPHER NORMENT

Oppenheimer Is Watching Me: A Memoir
JEFF PORTER

Great Expectation: A Father's Diary
DAN ROCHE

The Fluency of Light: Coming of Age in a Theater of Black and White
AISHA SABATINI SLOAN

Confessions of a Left-Handed Man: An Artist's Memoir
PETER SELGIN

The Harvard Black Rock Forest
GEORGE W. S. TROW

Detailing Trauma: A Poetic Anatomy
ARIANNE ZWARTJES